Telemedicine

A Practical Guide about the Benefits and Regulations of Telehealth for Medical Providers, Mental Health Professionals and Patients

Mike Richards

Copyright 2020 © Mike Richards.

ALL RIGHTS RESERVED. This book contains material protected under International and Federal Copyright Laws and Treaties. Any unauthorized reprint or use of this material is prohibited. No part of this book may be reproduced or transmitted in any form or by any means, electronic or mechanical, including photocopying, recording, or by any information storage and retrieval system without express written permission from the author/publisher.

Table of Contents

Introduction to Telehealth 12
Patient portal 14
Virtual appointments 15
Remote monitoring 16
Specialists talking to specialists 17
Individual health records 17
Personal health applications 18
The capability of telehealth 18
The limitations of telehealth 19

Chapter 1 20
Health and sustainable development 20
Ways Telehealth Is Taking Modern Healthcare to the Next Level 21

Chapter 2 26
Telehealth Use in Rural Healthcare 26
How does telehealth improve healthcare access in-country networks, and what kinds

of services have demonstrated to be compelling?... 27

What is the difference between telemedicine and telehealth? 31

How do Telehealth Resource Centers (TRCs) help country human services offices create telehealth benefits inside their association? 32

What are some telehealth financing programs for rural suppliers? 35

What are the challenges identified with telehealth benefits in rural communities? 36

Licensure 38

Broadband 40

What offices, technology, and staffing would our office need to actualize telehealth services? 41

In what capacity can telehealth be utilized to arrive at patients in their homes? 42

How does the utilization of telehealth impact rural healthcare suppliers? 44

What financial impact could the expansion of telehealth services have on a rural facility and community? 45

Is telehealth use across the board in rural facilities? 47

Chapter 3 50

Benefit and concerns for Telehealth practice 50

Pros of Telemedicine 50

Telemedicine Cost Effectiveness and Healthcare Savings 51

Expanded Specialist and Referring Physician Access 52

Expanded Patient Engagement 53

Better Patient Care Quality 53

Cons of Telemedicine 54

Specialized Training and Equipment 54

Reduced Care Continuity 54

Less In-Person Consultations 55

Precarious Policies and Reimbursement Rules 56

Chapter 4 57
Telehealth is a Service Delivery Model 57
Telehealth: A Service Delivery Model 59
Telehealth Reimbursement 60

Chapter 5 64
Laws and Regulations 64
What Is Telehealth? 64
Telehealth Licensing 65
Telehealth Reimbursement 67
Informed Consent 68
17 Best Telemedicine Companies 70

Chapter 6 80
Types of Telemedicine 80
Store-and-Forward Telemedicine 80
Remote Patient Monitoring 81
Real-time telemedicine 81
9 Myths of Telemedicine 82

Ways Telehealth Leads to Higher Patient Satisfaction Levels 88

Chapter 7 93
Building a Telehealth Program: Where Do I Start? 93
Discover Your Flag-Bearers 94
Support Hand-Raising 95
Enter the telehealth stage left. 96
Challenge the Status Quo 97

Chapter 8 100
How Much Does It Cost to Develop a Telemedicine App Like Doctor on Demand? 100
What is Doctor on Demand? 100
Why are telemedicine applications so popular? 101
Advantages that pull in patients 101
Advantages that pull in doctors 102
Highlights of a telemedicine application 103
Highlights for doctors 106

Electronic medical records 106

How telemedicine applications bring in cash 107

Difficulties of building up a telemedicine application 109

Chapter 9 112

Employment 112

What Are Telemedicine and Telehealth Jobs? 112

Basic Jobs and Who's Hiring 113

Telehealth Models for Promoting Workforce Recruitment and Retention ... 114

Instances of Recruitment and Retention through Telehealth 116

Implementation Considerations 118

Public Policy Implications 119

Tele-Emergency's Role in Connected Health 123

Significance of Sustainability Planning for Telehealth Programs 126

Maintainability Strategies for Rural Telehealth Programs 128

Repayment for Telehealth Services 129

Worth Based Payment Mechanisms 131

Telehealth User Fees 132

Working with Payers and Policymakers . 134

Award Funding for Telehealth Programs 136

Chapter 10 139

Telemedicine 139

1. History of Telemedicine 139

2. Telemedicine Today 143

3. The difference between telemedicine and telehealth 145

4. Telemedicine Pros and Cons 148

Experts of Telemedicine 149

More advantageous, available care for patients 149

Cons 152

5. Top Telemedicine Medical Specialties 155

6. What services can be given by telemedicine.. 159

7. How partners' telemedicine work/How would it be able to be utilized/Types of telemedicine...161

Remote patient observing....................... 166

Real-time telehealth 167

When to utilize telemedicine 170

Make an alternate course of action for crises and referrals................................... 172

Quiet Management and Evaluation 172

Quality Assurance................................... 174

Billing.. 175

Components that Affect Medicaid Reimbursement for Telemedicine 181

Chapter 11 189

Referrals and payment source 189

When referred patients denounce any authority 189

Conclusion...193

About Mike Richards................................195

Introduction to Telehealth

How often have you heard it said that the internet had changed present-day life? Surely it's most likely changed how you keep in contact with loved ones, buy goods and services, and even quest for information about medical issues.

An assortment of telehealth tools is accessible to assist you in dealing with your medicinal services and get the services you need. Is it accurate to say that you are exploiting them?

What is telehealth?

Telehealth is the utilization of digital information and correspondence technologies, for example, PCs and cell phones, to get to medicinal services benefits remotely and deal with your human services. These might be innovations you use from home or that your doctor uses to improve or bolster health care services.

Consider, for instance, the ways telehealth could support you if you have diabetes. You could do a few or the entirety of the accompanying:

- Utilize a cell phone or other device to transfer nourishment logs, meds, dosing, and blood sugar level for review by a medical caretaker who reacts electronically.

- Watch a video on carbohydrate counting and download an application for it to your telephone.
- Utilize an application to estimate, in light of your eating routine and exercise level, how much insulin you need.
- Utilize an online patient portal to see your test outcomes, schedule arrangements, demand medicine tops off, or email your doctor.
- Request testing supplies and drugs online.
- Get a portable retinal photoscreening at your doctor's office instead of planning a meeting with a specialist.
- Get email, text, or telephone updates when you need a flu shot, foot test, or other preventive consideration.

The objectives of telehealth, likewise called e-health or m-health (mobile health), incorporate the accompanying:

- Make human services open to individuals who live in rural or isolated communities.
- Make benefits all the more promptly accessible or advantageous for individuals with limited mobility, time, or transportation alternatives.
- Give access to a medical specialist.

- Improve correspondence and coordination of care among individuals from a human services group and a patient.

- Offer help for self-administration of human services.

The accompanying instances of telehealth services might be gainful for your health care.

Patient portal

Your essential consideration center may have an online patient portal. These entries offer a choice to email, which is a generally uncertain intends to impart about private medical information. An entrance gives an increasingly secure online tool to do the accompanying:

- Speak with your primary care physician or a medical caretaker.
- Solicitation medicine tops off.
- Audit test results and rundowns of past visits.
- Calendar arrangements or solicitation arrangement updates.

If your doctor is in a huge human services framework, the portal likewise may give a solitary purpose of correspondence for any specialist you may see.

Virtual appointments

A few clinics may give virtual arrangements that empower you to see your doctor or a medical attendant using online videoconferencing. These arrangements empower you to get progressing care from your standard specialist when an in-person visit isn't required or conceivable.

Other virtual arrangements incorporate online "visits" with a doctor or nurse practitioner. These services are, for the most part, for minor ailments, like the services accessible at a drop-in center. Some huge organizations give access to virtual specialists' workplaces as a piece of their health care offerings.

At the point when you sign into online assistance, you are guided through a progression of inquiries. The specialist or nurse practitioner can endorse meds, propose home consideration systems, or prescribe extra clinical care.

Thus, a nursing call focus is set up with medical attendants who utilize an inquiry and-answer configuration to give counsel to mind at home. A nursing call focus doesn't analyze an ailment or endorse drugs.

While these services are helpful, they have downsides:

- Treatment may not be composed of your standard specialist.

- Basic data from your clinical history may not be considered.
- The computer-driven decision making may not be ideal if you have a perplexing medical history.
- The virtual visit does not have an in-person assessment, which may hamper precise findings.
- The service doesn't effortlessly take into consideration doctor-patient decision making about medications or making an arrangement B if an underlying treatment doesn't work.

Remote monitoring

An assortment of innovations empowers your doctor or medicinal services group to screen your wellbeing remotely. These advancements include:

- Web-based or mobile apps for transferring data, for example, blood glucose readings, to your primary care physician or medicinal services group
- Devices that measure and remotely transmit data, for example, pulse, blood glucose or lung function
- Wearable devices that naturally record and transmit data, for example, pulse, blood glucose, step, pose control, tremors, physical action or sleep patterns

- Home observing devices for more seasoned individuals or individuals with dementia that recognize changes in ordinary exercises, for example, falls

Specialists talking to specialists

Specialists can likewise exploit innovation to give a better mind to their patients. One model is a virtual counsel that permits essential consideration specialists to get a contribution from pros when they have inquiries concerning your finding or treatment.

The essential consideration specialist sends test notes, history, test results, X-beams, or different pictures to the expert to review. The specialist may react electronically, direct a virtual meeting with you at your doctor's office, or request a face-to-face meeting.

These virtual counsels may forestall superfluous in-person referrals to a specialist, decrease hang tight times for specialist input and dispose of pointless travel.

Individual health records

An electronic individual wellbeing record framework — frequently called a PHR framework — is an assortment of data about your wellbeing that you control and keep up. A PHR application is available to you whenever using a web-empowered device, for example, your computer, laptop, tablet, or cell phone.

In a crisis, an individual wellbeing record can rapidly give emergency personnel vital information, for example, current analyses, prescriptions, drug allergies, and your doctor's contact information.

Personal health applications

A large number of applications have been made to assist purchasers with bettering arrange their medical information in one secure spot. These digital tools may support you:

- Store individual health information.
- Record vital signs.
- Compute and track caloric intake.
- Timetable updates for taking medication.
- Record physical action, for example, your day by day step count.

The capability of telehealth

Technology can improve the nature of health care and make it available to more individuals. Telehealth may give chances to make healthcare progressively effective, better planned, and closer to home.

Research about telehealth is still generally new; however, it's developing. For instance, a 2016 survey of studies found that both phone-based help and telemonitoring of imperative indications of individuals with cardiovascular breakdown diminished the risk of death and hospitalization for cardiovascular breakdown and improved personal satisfaction.

The limitations of telehealth

While telehealth has the potential for better-organized consideration, it likewise risks fragmenting health care. Fragmented care may prompt holes in care, abuse of clinical consideration, wrong utilization of meds, or unnecessary overlapping care.

The potential advantages of telehealth administrations might be restricted by different variables, for example, the capacity to pay for them. Insurance repayment for telehealth still differs by state and sort of protection. Likewise, a few people who might profit most from improved access to mind might be constrained as a result of regional internet availability or the expense of cell devices.

Chapter 1

Health and sustainable development

Telehealth includes the utilization of broadcast communications and virtual technology to convey healthcare outside of traditional medicinal services offices. Telehealth, which requires getting to just to telecommunications, is the essential component of "eHealth," which utilizes a more extensive scope of information and communication technologies (ICTs).

Telehealth models incorporate virtual home medicinal services, where patients, for example, the regularly sick or the old, may get direction in specific systems while staying at home. Telehealth has additionally made it simpler for health care workers in remote field settings to acquire direction from professionals somewhere else in the determination, care, and referral of patients. Preparing can sometimes additionally be conveyed using telehealth plans or with related technologies, for example, eHealth, which utilizes little computers and health.

Very much structured telehealth plans can improve healthcare access and results, especially for chronic disease treatment and for helpless groups. In addition to the fact that they reduce requests on packed offices, however, they likewise make cost savings and make the health sector more resilient.

Since remote communication and treatment of patients lessens the number of visits for health services, both transport-related emissions, and emissions identified with operational necessities is decreased. Likewise, fewer space requests can bring about littler wellbeing offices, with simultaneous decreases in construction materials, vitality and water utilization, waste, and overall environmental impacts.

Ways Telehealth Is Taking Modern Healthcare to the Next Level

At the point when he developed the phone, Alexander Graham Bell's first words to his assistant were: "Come here, Mr. Watson, I should see you." Legend has it that Bell brought his right hand over because the inventor had spilled acid on his pants and required medical attention; provided that this is true, it's one of the main known instances of telehealth.

The vast majority got mindful of telehealth during the 1980s. From that point forward, telehealth has developed to envelop a wide scope of devices and technologies that can transmit clinical data progressively around the world, permitting clinical experts to offer types of assistance to networks beforehand underserved. Further, it's being utilized all the more regularly for both open and private wellbeing suppliers the same, including for the treatment of mental illness, for example, depression, sparing lives in a crisis, and improving long term wellbeing results after a stroke.

1. Telehealth Brings Expertise to All Areas

The utilization of medical devices to screen a patient's wellbeing from a far distance presents another degree of comfort for both patient and supplier. It can serve to enhance face to face visits to a medical practitioner, and supplements ordinary specialist visits, making an increasingly complete treatment plan. Furthermore, it can give an extra mind that would somehow or another be inaccessible.

For instance, communities without a devoted stroke team may not realize how to oversee somebody amidst a stroke. With telehealth, they can talk with somebody who can assess the patient and ensure they get the correct course of treatment at the perfect time.

This won't wipe out visits to the specialist's office completely. Rather, telehealth and physical arrangements will work a couple with one another. The practitioner who reviews and screens the patient should know whether they are fulfilling the base guidelines they would need to think about a patient, remembering for individual visits appropriately. If not, the practitioner won't have enough information to help their medical management.

2. Telehealth Assists People with Limited Access to Specialized Care

The greatest advantage of telehealth is the capacity to give prompt access to mind that, in any case, would be hard to get. Rustic communities, for instance, do not have the medicinal services foundation of all the more thickly populated areas. Regularly, country patients need to drive hours to see a practitioner, which isn't constantly reasonable or conceivable. Telehealth makes an elective path for patients and professionals to stay in contact between arrangements or for patients to have visits with specialists that they would usually not have the option to have.

What's more, communities cut off by tornadoes, typhoons, and another natural disaster can use telehealth for extra basic consideration get to. In ongoing debacles, trauma doctors, nervous system specialists, and other strength suppliers have had the option to Skype in to talk with individuals on the ground in the disaster area. This permitted them to offer particular types of assistance where they wouldn't have, in any case, had the option to get them and spares experience that could have been lost.

3. Telehealth Is Practical and Relatively Inexpensive for Patients

There is a declining misconception that, since it speaks to advance technology, telehealth is additionally restrictively costly. Previously, suppliers were seldom repaid for telehealth services, so those services struggled to pick up footing. While this has verifiably been a boundary in telehealth, it's quickly improving. More medical coverage organizations, alongside Medicaid and Medicare, are repaying the utilization of telehealth. Subsequently, patients see it as an increasingly practical, dependable framework.

What's more, wearable devices like Fitbits and Apple Watches, which are in the telehealth classification, can be bought by the general shopper for a few hundred dollars or less. Those devices can likewise be helpful for some reasons, from patients endeavoring to lose undesirable weight, to checking constant wellbeing conditions, which eventually decreases future patient costs.

4. Telehealth Maximizes Access to Mental Health Care

One zone profiting most from the utilization of telehealth is mental health care. Checking visits for regular mental health struggle, for example, depression or nervousness, use little hands-on physical appraisal and have more to do with talking with the patient.

By exploiting telehealth using video communication, patients can get a brisk 10-minute conference, lighten a prompt issue that perhaps would have spiraled into something progressively huge, get a remedy and go to standard treatment meetings. Numerous insurance agencies offer emotional wellness care through video calls, and numerous free associations offer virtual choices.

5. Telehealth's Benefits Set to Grow

Everybody who utilizes the medicinal services industry will have a treatment plan that incorporates telehealth in some style, regardless of whether through remote visits with a primary care provider, or progressively extensive care, for example, seeing an advisor all the time. As insurance agencies pattern toward repaying more telehealth treatment options, telehealth will just keep on developing increasingly across the widespread and advantageous, helping increment the general wellbeing and prosperity of urban and rustic communities the same. The fate of healthcare is indivisible from telehealth.

Chapter 2

Telehealth Use in Rural Healthcare

Telehealth can help healthcare frameworks, associations, and suppliers grow access to and improve the nature of country human services. Utilizing telehealth in country regions to convey and help with the delivery of healthcare services can lessen or limit difficulties and weights patients experience, for example, transportation issues identified with going for a claim to fame care. Telehealth can likewise improve observing, practicality, and correspondences inside the healthcare framework.

Telehealth utilizes telecommunications technology and other electronic data to help with clinical human healthcare services gave a good ways off, which can likewise incorporate giving education, authoritative capacities, and peer meetings. While one of the most widely recognized pictures of telehealth is that of a patient talking by videoconference with a human services provider who is found remotely, telehealth can take different structures, including:

- Remote patient monitoring (RPM)
- Store and forward transmission of medical information
- Mobile health communication (mHealth)

This guide gives an overview of telehealth in provincial America to help medicinal services suppliers discover data identified by giving telehealth services and features subsidizing openings and different activities to execute telehealth services. The guide incorporates instances of telehealth ventures to fill in as models for rustic emergency clinics and facilities to create and execute telehealth programs. Difficulties for giving telehealth benefits in rustic regions are additionally examined, for example, workforce issues, nature of care concerns, repayment, licensure, and access to broadband administrations.

How does telehealth improve healthcare access in-country networks, and what kinds of services have demonstrated to be compelling?

The National Academies of Science, Engineering, and Medicine 2012 workshop summary, The Role of Telehealth in an Evolving Health Care Environment, talks about how telehealth can drive volume, increment the nature of human services, and decrease generally costs by diminishing readmissions and avoidable crisis office visits for rustic networks. Telehealth permits small rural hospitals to give quality healthcare services at lower costs and in the neighborhood human services office, which benefits provincial patients since they are never again required to venture out significant distances to get to claim to fame care. Staying away from persistent exchanges when care can be given locally is basic to both little clinic and supplier practicality in provincial regions. It likewise assists tertiary with caring focuses keep beds open for patients needing critical care.

Utilizing telehealth to give specialty service is more attainable for rural medicinal services offices than setting up those country offices with strength and subspecialty suppliers. Telehealth permits specialists and subspecialists to visit rural patients for all intents and purposes, improving access just as making a more extensive scope of healthcare services accessible to rural communities using telemedicine, including:

- Radiology
- Psychiatry
- Ophthalmology
- Dermatology
- Dentistry
- Audiology
- Cardiology
- Oncology
- Obstetrics

Frequently, rural primary care providers and subspecialist suppliers can fill in as a group to share information and oversee quiet consideration through the e-counsel model or other effective projects, for example, Project ECHO® – Extension for Community Healthcare Outcomes. Successful healthcare services and projects managed through telehealth innovation in rural communities include:

- **Chronic care management intercessions are** utilizing telehealth to give patients access to incorporated consideration during their primary care visits.
- Access to **emergency care** suppliers continuously for assessments and counsels to neighborhood suppliers. Avera eCARE Emergency gives emergency consultations and a variety of emergency services using telehealth to rural emergency rooms.
- **Home monitoring** can connect with patients in their homes between medical visits by helping them viably deal with their conditions. Bridges to Care Transitions-Remote Home Monitoring and Chronic Disease Self-Management is an example of a telehealth remote monitoring program that helps patients with chronic disease management and behavioral health conditions in their homes.

- **Intensive care units (ICUs)** give around the clock critical care observing by a group of subspecialists and critical care nurses. Avera eCARE ICU gives every minute of every day concentrated consideration checking of fundamentally sick patients using telehealth.
- **Long term care** services offered through telehealth can carry specific consideration to old populaces who live in long term care offices in rural areas. Telehealth technology, actualized in the SD residential Facilities Healthcare Services Access Project, permits authorities situated in urban regions to associate with residents in-country long term care offices with chronic health problems.

- **Online therapy and remote counseling** join rural residents with urban social wellbeing and emotional well-being counseling services. In Texas, the Madison Outreach and Services through Telehealth (MOST) Network offers to direct administrations by video and telephone to Spanish-talking inhabitants.
- **Telepharmacy** stretches out access to pharmacy services, including meds and medicine counseling, at rural healthcare facilities and communities' pharmacies.

- Electronic correspondences interface suppliers are working in confined territories to make **visual professional communities** that can help with patient care.
- Human services suppliers' utilization of cell phones, for example, tablets and cell phones, can improve interchanges with patients and different suppliers.
- Interpreter services can be transmitted on-request through sound as well as visual innovation for patients who talk restricted or no English.

Programs supported by telehealth offer new techniques for improving health care access and quality by broadening the compass of human services, improving the capacity of rural suppliers to address a more extensive scope of ailments, and encouraging coordinated effort between professionals with restricted access to their partners.

What is the difference between telemedicine and telehealth?

The Health Resources and Services Administration's (HRSA) Office for the Advancement of Telehealth (OAT) characterizes telehealth as:

utilizing electronic information and broadcast communications technologies to help significant distance clinical human services, patient and expert wellbeing related training, general wellbeing, and health administration.

The Office of the National Coordinator for Health Information Technology's (ONC) Health IT Playbook characterizes telemedicine as remote clinical services with intuitive wellbeing interchanges with clinicians on the two parts of the bargains.

Telehealth can incorporate remote non-clinical services, for example, preparing, Project ECHO®, administrative meetings, and proceeding with clinical training, notwithstanding clinical services. Although telehealth is more extensive in scope, the American Telemedicine Association and numerous different associations utilize the terms telemedicine and telehealth reciprocally.

How do Telehealth Resource Centers (TRCs) help country human services offices create telehealth benefits inside their association?

The 12 provincial and 2 national TRCs make up the National Consortium of Telehealth Resource Centers (NCTRC). They are financed by Office for the Advancement of Telehealth (OAT) to help healthcare associations, systems, and suppliers with executing and addressing continuous inquiries identified with practical telehealth projects to serve rustic and restoratively underserved zones and populaces. The national TRCs are:

- Centre for Connected Health Policy: The National Telehealth Policy Resource Center (CCHP)
- National Telehealth Technology Assessment Resource Center (TTAC)

The regional TRCs comprise of:

California Telehealth Resource Center (CTRC)

Great Plains Telehealth Resource and Assistance Center (gpTRAC)

Heartland Telehealth Resource Center (HTRC)

Mid-Atlantic Telehealth Resource Center (MATRC)

Upper east Telehealth Resource Center (NETRC)

Northwest Regional Telehealth Resource Center (NRTRC)

Pacific Basin Telehealth Resource Center (PBTRC)

South Central Telehealth Resource Center (SCTRC)

Southeastern Telehealth Resource Center (SETRC)

Southwest Telehealth Resource Center (SWTRC)

TexLa Telehealth Resource Center (TexLa)

Upper Midwest Regional Telehealth Resource Center (UMTRC)

To locate the regional TRC that serves your state, see NCTRC's Find Your TRC map and select on your state. NCTRC offers actuality sheets; aides, layouts, and checklists; research catalogs; news; events; and online courses that spread a wide scope of subjects including:

- Staffing and enrolling specialists
- Instruction and training
- Credentialing and permitting
- Medical malpractice and obligation
- Repayment
- Billing
- Evaluation
- Advertising

Telehealth Connect is a registry to find telehealth provider sites in the U.S. that can be looked at by clinical strength, area, practice type, and more. NCTRC has a national TRC webinar series that offers month to month online courses on telehealth and related themes. Past online courses in the arrangement are additionally accessible as resources.

What are some telehealth financing programs for rural suppliers?

There are a few award programs concentrated on funding rural telehealth projects:

The U.S. Department of Agriculture (USDA) Rural Development supports a few projects and opportunities for telehealth:

- o Rustic Broadband Access Loan and Loan Guarantee Program gives assets to the expenses of development, improvement, or securing of offices and equipment expected to offer broadband assistance in qualified provincial zones.
- o USDA Distance Learning and Telemedicine Loan and Grant Program offer awards to help and improve telemedicine and separation learning services in country regions.
- o USDA Community Facilities Direct Loan and Grant Program grants direct credits and additionally gives for essential community facilities in rural areas.
- The Telehealth Network Grant Program (TNGP) is offered by the Federal Office of Rural Health Policy. TNGP gives subsidizing to telehealth networks and programs to improve access to healthcare benefits in rural, frontiers, and underserved regions.

- The Universal Service Administrative Company (USAC) offers the Rural Health Care Telecommunications Program that gives help to country healthcare suppliers on qualified costs for broadband and media communications get to.

Extra subsidizing for country telehealth projects and opportunities can be found in the Funding and Opportunities area of this guide.

What are the challenges identified with telehealth benefits in rural communities?

Notwithstanding the guarantee telehealth holds for improving access to healthcare benefits in rural areas, there are regularly strategy obstructions and infrastructure insufficiencies that must be survived. A few difficulties to telehealth reception, implementation, and achievement include:

Reimbursement

The issue of Medicare repayment is usually referred to as a significant challenge for telehealth programs. CCHP's 2019 fact sheet, Telehealth Reimbursement, examines a few reactions of the present Medicare reimbursement model for telehealth including:

- Geographic and starting site restrictions
- Supplier restrictions

- Service restrictions

Individual state Medicaid programs change in their rules concerning reimbursement for telehealth services. CCHP's 2019 report, State Telehealth Laws and Reimbursement Policies, outlines telehealth-related laws and repayment approaches for every one of the 50 states and the District of Columbia. The report remembers a concentration for Medicaid inclusion for telehealth. CCHP likewise keeps up two intelligent maps, one for current telehealth state laws and repayment approaches and the other for telehealth enactment and guideline following. The National Rural Health Association (NRHA) strategy brief, 2017 Telehealth Policy for the National Rural Health Association, explains on hindrances to telehealth and gives approach proposals to expand access to telehealth. Reimbursement by private payers for telehealth administrations can likewise shift. Some health insurance organizations repay for telehealth administrations, while others don't.

The Center for Telehealth and e-Health Law (CTeL) attempts to address the legal and regulatory barriers to the selection of telehealth. CTeL gives a Reimbursement Overview of telehealth and spreads Medicare Reimbursement and Medicaid Reimbursement more inside and out.

Licensure

The 2013 NRHA strategy brief, Streamlining Telemedicine Licensure to Improve Rural America, portrays how the present doctor licensure framework places loads on doctors needing to grow their training to rustic territories. Doctors who wish to rehearse across state lines must be authorized by the expert permitting board in each state where they are conveying care to patients. Telehealth and Licensing Interstate Providers, a National Conference of State Legislatures 2016 preparation paper, investigates moves states have made to ease licensure boundaries and the related weight, for example,

- Offering explicit licenses for telehealth
- Reciprocity and underwriting with different states
- Making interstate compacts

The Interstate Medical Licensure Compact (IMLC) is an understanding between 29 states, the District of Columbia, and the domain of Guam, and 43 osteopathic and clinical sheets inside those states and region that offers a sped-up process for qualified doctors to be authorized to practice in various states. For more information on the procedure, capabilities, and the agreement, see IMLC's every sometimes posed question. The U.S. Department of Veterans Affairs (VA) is a special case; VA doctors have license movability that permits them to practice across state lines to any place the patient is accepting care.

There are numerous other licensure compacts engaged with the delivery of healthcare services to rural populations utilizing telehealth, including:

- Psychology Interjurisdictional Compact (PSYPACT)
- Nurse Licensure Compact (NLC)
- Advanced Practice Registered Nurse Compact (APRN Compact)
- Physical therapy Licensure Compact

A 2015 report from the American Hospital Association (AHA), Realizing the Promise of Telehealth: Understanding the Legal and Regulatory Challenges, covers difficulties suppliers experience while giving patient consideration utilizing telehealth, for example, coverage and payment issues, licensure, credentialing, privileging, online endorsing, privacy and security concerns, misbehavior and risk protection, and that's just the beginning. The report offers strategy contemplations to address telehealth barriers, including:

- Exhaustive payment approaches
- Setting measures for the advancement of clinical guidelines and protocols

- Organizing state laws to help shared objectives concerning doctor licensure portability

Broadband

Affordable broadband is required to help telehealth programs, health information technology (HIT), and health information exchanges (HIEs), all of which increment access to and the nature of medicinal services. Numerous rural communities don't as of now approaching web association speeds, which supports the powerful and effective transmission of information to give telehealth services.

Extra difficulties limiting the reception of telehealth in rural areas, including malpractice, HIPAA and protection, security, endorsing, and credentialing, are talked about in CCHP's 2019 Telehealth Policy Barriers fact sheet. Rural broadband access and its significance is clarified further in RHIhub's Health Information Technology in Rural Healthcare topic guide question Why is broadband significant for HIT? How might we tell if broadband is accessible in our community?

What offices, technology, and staffing would our office need to actualize telehealth services?

While technology issues, for example, pattern availability and interoperability, can affect telehealth execution, fruitful projects understand that the innovation must be actualized in the correct procedures to get the best results.

A few contemplations include:

- Services to be upheld and upgraded through telehealth
- Installment models and reimbursement
- Equipment required, which can shift and is reliant on kind of services to be given
- Proper facilities for technology where administrations are to be given
- Data management services for dealing with, putting away, printing, and transmitting medical information
- Preparing of suppliers and staff
- Supplier and staff purchase in
- Support staff to execute telehealth programs
- Protection and security concerns

California Telehealth Resource Center (CTRC) built up a Telehealth Coordinator Online Training that spreads significant ideas and assets expected to assemble an information base and the aptitudes fundamental for a telehealth organizer. If you might want help with new or existing telehealth services or if you have explicit inquiries in regards to your office, contact your regionalTRC.

In what capacity can telehealth be utilized to arrive at patients in their homes?

Remote patient monitoring (RPM) can be utilized to arrive at patients in their homes. RPM is the assortment of personal health and medical data from patients in their homes. After data collection, the data are transmitted to a human services supplier in an alternate area to be utilized in healthcare decision making. Some RPM program models include:

- Extensions to Care Transitions-Remote Home Monitoring and Chronic Disease Self-Management is a joint effort between three healthcare associations that attempt to recognize and enlist in risk patients in an RPM program and a constant illness instruction and training program after an inpatient hospitalization or crisis room visit.
- Intermountain Healthcare Connect Care Pro®, offers access to healthcare for rural communities through 35 telehealth benefits in three different ways: clinician-to-clinician, direct-to-customer, and RPM. Connect Care Pro® has existing projects for hypertension

and diabetes; however, it is creating RPM programs for chronic obstructive pulmonary disease (COPD), movement, and health.

Mobile health can be utilized by suppliers and general wellbeing units to speak with patients and residents in their homes. mHealth is the utilization of cell phones to give wellbeing related data, which can incorporate general instruction, exceptional notices, or correspondence through a wellbeing application. mHealth can likewise be utilized for remote observing, where individual wellbeing and clinical information are gathered from a patient in his home. The Rise of mHealth reports that cell phones, applications, tablets, and other smart devices are turning into a necessary piece of mHealth. National Telehealth Technology Assessment Resource Center (TTAC) offers an overview of mHealth innovation and different assets identified with product information and product assessment.

Telecare is a term for offering remote monitoring to individuals who are old or have incapacities. Telecare gives care and observation to permit these patients to live autonomously in their homes.

How does the utilization of telehealth impact rural healthcare suppliers?

A 2015 National Advisory Committee on Rural Health and Human Services approach brief, Telehealth in Rural America, examines how telehealth use in country regions can lessen a supplier's sentiments of segregation and burn out, and in this way, improve supplier maintenance at a rural hospital.

Telemedicine: Changing the Landscape of Rural Physician Practice, features tributes from medicinal services suppliers rehearsing in rural areas all through the U.S. Dr. Wilbur Hitt talks about his encounters of how telehealth diminishes provincial practice segregation:

Telemedicine cultivates a coordinated effort that lessens the sentiments of detachment that doctors may encounter when they go to practice in a small town. With telemedicine, it resembles having one foot in the city, however, having the option to live and rehearse out in a rural area. It's likewise consoling to realize that you're destined for success with the treatment plan and are remaining current.

Healthcare systems with the foundation and staffing to help telehealth services sway how rural suppliers can give patient care by giving them access to:

- Group-based care
- Different specialists and subspecialists for counsels progressively
- Virtual networks with peers
- Outsourced indicative investigations
- In-home checking of patients for follow-up care
- Proceeding with instruction and training, diminishing travel and out-of-practice time

Executing telehealth requires staff preparation and changes in work processes, arrangements, and techniques. NCTRC offers telehealth assets and tools for doctors and other healthcare staff.

What financial impact could the expansion of telehealth services have on a rural facility and community?

The budgetary effect of actualizing telehealth benefits in a community can shift, contingent upon the kind of healthcare service or services to be offered to utilize telehealth and the patient populace. The 2017 NTCA: The Rural Broadband Association report, Anticipating Economic Returns of Rural Telehealth, portrays potential telehealth advantages including the accompanying quantifiable advantages:

- Transportation costs

- Lost wages
- Clinic staffing costs
- Local lab and drug store benefits

The report likewise records nonquantifiable benefits:

- Access to experts
- Opportune consideration
- Comfort
- Transportation
- Advantages to the supplier
- Improved patient results

Furthermore, more states have begun to consider enactment, for example, telehealth parity laws, which would expect back up plans to cover services gave using telehealth technology at a similar rate concerning services conveyed face to face. A guide on the American Telemedicine Association's site shows which states have equality laws, halfway equality laws, and proposed equality law enactment for private insurance coverage of telemedicine.

Hospitals that utilization teleconsultation and telementoring services can hold income when suppliers at those medical clinics can treat patients in a nearby healthcare office, rather than moving to another medicinal services office for specialty care.

A 2011 report, Estimating the Economic Impact of Telemedicine in a Rural Community, portrays an investigation of 24 hospitals in four Midwestern states with enormous rural areas: Kansas, Oklahoma, Arkansas, and Texas. All medical clinics inside these communities practice some type of telemedicine. The aftereffects of the investigation decided:

- Every people group distinguished yearly reserve funds or another economic opportunity of $20,000 or more.
- The normal yearly financial effect for a network was evaluated at $522,000, with a most extreme effect of more than $1,300,000.
- Most of the investment funds exhibited originated from the privately performed lab and pharmacy services.

Is telehealth use across the board in rural facilities?

A 2019 American Hospital Association (AHA) publication, Fact Sheet: Telehealth, found a predictable positive pattern in the number of emergency clinics utilizing telehealth services. In 2010, 35% of hospitals announced full or incomplete execution that developed to 76% of medical clinics detailing telehealth use in 2017. Utilization of Telemedicine among Rural Medicare Beneficiaries discovered telemedicine visits for country Medicare recipients expanded from 2004 to 2013 at a yearly development pace of 28%. The article reports almost 80% of rural beneficiary telehealth visits were for emotional wellness conditions.

A 2014 RUPRI Center for Rural Health Policy Analysis report, Extent of Telehealth Use in Rural and Urban Hospitals, talked about key discoveries from an investigation of medical clinic based telehealth utilization and found:

- Only 33% of rural hospitals in the examination gave some telehealth services. The other 66% of the rural hospitals either didn't give telehealth benefits or were in the first place phases of actualizing telehealth services.
- Hospitals distinguished as scholastic clinical focuses, not-for-benefits, or medical clinics partnered with a bigger human services framework were bound to have some type of telehealth.
- Rural and urban medical clinics actualized telehealth at comparable rates.
- Rural medical clinics were bound to utilize telehealth to help with giving radiology, crisis, and trauma healthcare services.
- Urban hospitals were bound to utilize telehealth for some specialties and subspecialties, including cardiology, stroke and coronary episode care, neurology,

obstetrics, gynecology, neonatal intensive care unit (NICU), and pediatrics.

Chapter 3

Benefits and concerns for Telehealth practice

It is safe to say that you are prepared to redesign your association to fuse telemedicine? Over a portion of all U.S. medical clinics use telemedicine, and this pattern is rising.

Indeed, in an ongoing overview of human services, officials discovered 90% had just started creating or actualizing a telemedicine program into their associations. Indeed, even healthcare suppliers in littler, independent practices are beginning to receive telehealth to contend with nearby retail facilities and quit losing their patients.

While the telemedicine business is developing, there are as yet a couple of difficulties to consider. Adding new advances and procedures to your association is a major move and shouldn't be messed with. This traces the advantages and disadvantages of telemedicine that you ought to consider before concluding whether to redesign your patient service.

Pros of Telemedicine

Receiving the most recent telemedicine activities can enable your training to accomplish various advantages. You can bring down healthcare costs, drive up proficiency and income, give your patients better access to medicinal services, and at last, get more joyful, more advantageous patients who remain in your association.

Progressively Convenient and Accessible Patient Care

As per an ongoing Cisco worldwide overview, 74% of patients incline toward simple access to medicinal services benefits over the face to face collaborations with suppliers.

In the present healthcare world, accommodation is vital.

Adding virtual care to your training offers patients straightforward, on-request care – without the typical sat around idly and cost of most face to face visits. Patients who live in remote areas, or who are homebound or can't take off time from work, can get to mind. Video conferencing, cell phone applications, and online services frameworks interface more patients with suppliers than at any time in recent memory.

Telemedicine Cost Effectiveness and Healthcare Savings

Remote examination and observing administrations and electronic information stockpiling healthcare service costs fundamentally, setting aside cash for you, your patients, and insurance agencies. Telemedicine likewise decreases pointless non-urgent ER visits and disposes of transportation costs for regular checkups.

As of late, the American Hospital Association investigated a telemedicine program that spared 11% in expenses and dramatically multiplied ROI for investors.

Past these general cost-investment funds, telehealth can help support income by transforming available to come into work hours into billable time, drawing in new patients, diminishing no-appears, and in any event, lessening overhead for doctors who choose to change to an adaptable work-from-home model for part of the week.

Expanded Specialist and Referring Physician Access

With telehealth, patients in country or remote zones profit by snappier and progressively advantageous authority get to. In the U.S., for every100,000 country patients, there are just 43 specialists accessible. These patients persevere through longer arrangement drives and experience difficulty getting to lifesaving discussions for explicit ailments or chronic care plans.

Telemedicine offers better access to more experts. You can allude your patients to the particular doctors they need, paying little mind to area.

Expanded Patient Engagement

At the point when patients are focused on their own human services goals, it prompts lower costs and improved wellbeing. Ernst and Young Senior Advisory Services Manager Jan Oldenburg disclosed to Healthcare IT News that "[t]he significant expense of separated purchasers influences everyone."

Connecting with your patients through telemedicine can assist them in keeping up arrangements and care plans. Expanded commitment activities can likewise check stoutness rates and tobacco use by helping you to empower your patients' sound way of life decisions.

Not exclusively do virtual visits promise patients that their suppliers are accessible and associated with their consideration, it makes it a lot simpler for them to connect with questions, report early admonition signs, and cause a to catch up an arrangement to ensure they're on target.

Better Patient Care Quality

Telemedicine offers understanding focused methodologies, for example, improved practicality of care. This is basic to quality patient consideration. Patients can address healthcare issues rapidly with continuous critical consideration meetings and find out about treatment choices in no time.

Another examination shows that telemedicine patients score lower for sorrow, tension, and stress, and have 38% less emergency clinic affirmations.

Cons of Telemedicine

While telemedicine vows to become quickly throughout the following decade and has clear advantages, it despite everything represents some specialized and viable issues for human services suppliers.

Specialized Training and Equipment

Rebuilding IT staff obligations and buying hardware requires significant investment and costs cash. Preparing is pivotal to building a powerful telemedicine program. Doctors, practice chiefs, and other clinical staff should be prepared on the new frameworks to guarantee a strong ROI. What's more, your staffing necessities may diminish. For example, a medical caretaker in a provincial Alaska office can screen up to 33 patients without a moment's delay from a solitary area utilizing telemedicine administrations.

Reduced Care Continuity

In situations where patients are utilizing on-request telemedicine services that associate them with an arbitrary human services supplier, care progression endures. A patient's essential care supplier might not approach records from those different visits and end up with an inadequate history for the patient. Specialist co-op rearranging builds the hazard that a specialist won't know a patient's history or have notes about consideration schedules.

Since reduced care progression can diminish care quality, traditional telemedicine suppliers must apply sound information answers to keep up satisfactory and open patient records. As more human services suppliers receive telehealth answers for use with their patients, care congruity will probably expand, decreasing the opportunity that patients end up at a retail facility or dire care place when they need speedy care.

Less In-Person Consultations

Stressed over technology's restrictions? You're not the only one. Numerous suppliers stress over specialized issues related to telemedicine. Senior Healthcare Group Consultant Arun Ravi revealed to Becker's Hospital Review that poor broadband associations could prompt "possible patient mismanagement."

Numerous suppliers and patients the same despite everything like an "individual touch," and not all strategies – even straightforward tests – can be performed carefully. Be that as it may, in situations where patients can't get in to see their doctors face to face, and for some cases that don't require a physical test, telehealth can be a good other option.

Precarious Policies and Reimbursement Rules

Healthcare laws, repayment strategies, and security assurance rules battle to stay aware of this quickly developing industry. As a healthcare supplier, you need to advance prescribed procedures when drawing nearer telemedicine.

While significant advancements have been made to telehealth repayment over the past couple of years, despite everything stays a typical hindrance for suppliers intrigued by telemedicine. It's ideal to do a little investigation into the repayment arrangement scene in your state (papers, articles, and so on.) before you begin.

What's Next?

Telemedicine is a $17.8 billion industry, and it's relied upon to become 18.4% every year from 2015–2020. While despite everything that has a few restrictions, numerous human services suppliers are developing to fathom these issues and improve their patients' entrance to quality care. Since you know a few weaknesses and advantages of telemedicine, you're prepared to begin pondering how your training will move toward this booming healthcare pattern.

Chapter 4

Telehealth is a Service Delivery Model

It is progressively apparent that telehealth can improve access to recovery services and specialists, forestall superfluous deferrals in accepting care, including climate occasions affecting travel and encourage facilitated care and interprofessional cooperation. The World Health Organization (WHO) certifies the adequacy of telehealth as a successful help delivery model for restoration experts (i.e., telerehabilitation). The WHO and World Bank, in their co-created World Report on Disability, audited explore on the utilization of telehealth to offer types of assistance for emotional wellness, heart recovery, remote evaluation for home alterations, discussion for prosthetics, orthotics, and wheelchair solution, and intellectual restoration among different services and closed: "Developing proof on the viability and adequacy of telerehabilitation shows that telerehabilitation prompts comparative or better clinical results when contrasted with conventional intercessions."

Research bolsters the utilization of telehealth as a service delivery model in occupational therapy. The AOTA Telehealth position is a convincing examination in the areas of wheelchair solution, neurological appraisal, versatile equipment prescription, and home alteration, ergonomic evaluation, school-based practice, early mediation administrations, wellbeing and health programming, and recovery for people who have encountered stroke, bosom malignant growth, horrible cerebrum injury, polytrauma, Parkinson's ailment, and other neurological and orthopedic debilitations.

A few similar adequacies concentrates likewise reason that there is no huge distinction in clinical results between occupational therapy services gave face to face and services gave through telehealth to wheelchair appraisal, pre-affirmation orthopedic word related treatment home visits, evaluation of exercises of day by day living and handwork in people with Parkinson's sickness and ergonomic appraisal. Also, high fulfillment among administration beneficiaries is accounted for.

Studies propose that with certain populaces and mediations, telehealth may bring about preferable results over the face to face benefits. In their survey of telehealth writing for emotional wellness and substance misuse, distinguished smoking end as one region where telehealth yielded preferable results over other options (e.g., face to face) approaches. Utilizing a solitary contextual investigation with exchanging treatment structure with benchmark and follow-up conditions, looked at the degree of autonomy of grown-ups with scholarly inabilities living in incorporated network settings observing standard consideration and telecare (i.e., telehealth). The utilization of telehealth brought about members finishing novel family unit exercises with more noteworthy freedom than the in-person treatment condition; be that as it may, the scientists advised against overgeneralization of the outcomes.

Intercessions that require physical taking care of or potentially understanding of unobtrusive body or logical signs may not be as powerful when conveyed through telehealth technologies. Be that as it may, even 'hands-on' petitions (e.g., Neuro-Developmental Treatment or NDT) can be upheld through telehealth by utilizing a consultative methodology between a specialist and novice practitioner.

Current telehealth proof is empowering, however, constrained. Further research is expected to figure out which OT evaluations and intercessions are manageable to a telehealth service delivery model.

Telehealth: A Service Delivery Model

It is imperative to perceive that telehealth is a service delivery model that is utilized to convey help, for example, OT. Telehealth can't particular and separate mediation. Consequently, the utilization of telehealth is inside the domain of existing word related treatment extents of training.

All prerequisites to hold fast to state, government, and moral rules for OT service delivery are similar to whether services are given face to face or through telehealth technologies. While numerous licensure sheets have embraced AOTA's situation on the utilization of telehealth, telehealth guidelines and arrangements regularly vary between states. It is along these lines officeholder upon an expert to decide whether there are prescriptive telehealth laws, guidelines, or strategies in the state wherein the professional is situated at the hour of administration, and (if unique) the state wherein the customer is situated at the hour of services.

Technologies and software utilized for the conveyance of OT services using telehealth must meet the Health Insurance Portability and Accountability Act and the Health Information Technology for Economic and Clinical Health Act (HITECH) prerequisites for security, security, and privacy of protected health information (PHI). Risk examination resources, including a list to dissect business video conferencing programming, can educate experts' consistency with HIPAA and HITECH necessities for protection, security, and secrecy of PHI.

Telehealth Reimbursement

Despite AOTA's attestation that "OT services furnished with telehealth advances ought to be esteemed, perceived, and repaid equivalent to administrations gave face to face," repayment for telehealth, while promising, can't widespread.

Positive patterns toward reimbursement incorporate the accompanying. Telehealth reimbursement is extending with authoritative commands for inclusion by private protection in 22 states at the hour of this composition (American Telemedicine Association; ATA,). Now and again, legally binding courses of action and private compensation are wellsprings of repayment for OT administrations gave through telehealth. The Department of Defense (U.S. Branch of Defense, 2014) and Veterans Health Administration have fundamentally extended its programming and money related help for telehealth. The Patient Protection and Affordable Care Act made open doors for consideration of telehealth in creative assistance conveyance and installment models; in any case, training and support is required for full incorporation of OT in these novel facilitated care and service delivery model.

Regardless of these advances, telehealth repayment can't. The Center for Medicare and Medicaid Services (CMS) Telehealth Provider List does exclude OT professionals (nor other restoration suppliers) as repaid 'telehealth suppliers' for Medicare recipients. Medicaid repayment despite everything fluctuates by state. For instance, Kentucky and New Mexico's Medicaid programs as of now repay OT, physical therapy (PT), and speech-language pathology (SLP) service delivery through telehealth. Interestingly, Virginia and Ohio have arrangements for SLP service delivered using telehealth administrations; however, not for telehealth conveyed OT or PT services. AOTA is working together with professionals and partners to advocate for extended repayment of OT services gave using telehealth.

InterState Practice And Telehealth

Except for clinical practice inside the federal care system, experts must hold an expert permit in the state wherein the customer is found. The advantages of telehealth can't be completely acknowledged except if suppliers can practice across state lines without any difficulty, maybe using interstate permit versatility or another methodology that can encourage improved access.

There are numerous potential advantages of interstate permit convey ability. Customers, paying little heed to geographic area, would appreciate more noteworthy straightforward entry to experts. State governments could lessen duplicative procedures and regulatory costs, maybe redistributing assets to reinforce purchaser assurance. Specialists may encounter fewer postponements, cost, and exertion related to acquiring, keeping up, and restoring numerous state licenses.

The exploration that follows gives models of how interstate practice benefits customers with complex ailments that require specific clinical management.

Chapter 5

Laws and Regulations

Patients today are progressively ready to utilize virtual consideration and telehealth services, mostly due to the comfort and capacity to improve access to human services. As indicated by a 2017 Virtual Visits Consumer Choice Survey from the Advisory Board, 77% of customers would consider seeing a healthcare provider. Almost one of every five – 19% – had just observed a supplier practically.

In any case, the law hasn't made up for lost time to the innovation despite the developing enthusiasm for telehealth. States have their laws around telehealth permitting, repayment and consent, just as their definitions for what comprises telehealth. It is significant for patients and healthcare suppliers to know about the laws in their state before utilizing telehealth services.

What Is Telehealth?

There is no standard definition for telehealth. However, it is extensively characterized as the utilization of electronic and media communications advancements to convey human clinical services administrations, persistent training, general health, and health organization. It is frequently utilized reciprocally with telemedicine; however, the last commonly centers around the act of medication through remote methods. Telehealth incorporates video conferencing, remote patient observation, and store-and-forward. Versatile wellbeing (mHealth) can cover with telehealth, yet the two can't be utilized conversely because mHealth is conveyed only using cell phones, for example, cell phones and tablets.

Telehealth Licensing

Permitting for telehealth differs from state to state. As indicated by HealthIT.gov, most states expect doctors to be authorized to rehearse in the beginning site's state. In contrast, others require the human services supplier to have a legitimate permit in the state where the patient is found. At the end of the day, if the healthcare supplier is situated in Arizona, however, the patient is situated in Maine, the supplier must have a substantial permit in Maine.

However, progress is being made toward permitting doctors to rehearse in various states. The Interstate Medical Licensure Compact (IMLC) is an understanding between 29 expresses, the District of Columbia, and the area of Guam that permits authorized doctors to rehearse medication across state lines inside the Compact if they meet certain settled upon qualification prerequisites. The Compact speeds up the application procedure by utilizing a doctor's current data from the state of principal license (SPL).

However, not all states are a piece of the IMLC yet. For instance, Minnesota received an enactment to enter the Compact in 2015. However, it should pass two new bills to meet new government law authorization personal investigations necessities, as indicated by the Minnesota Medical Association. New Jersey presented Compact enactment in May 2019 however can't part state yet.

Peruse here to become familiar with the IMLC part expresses that are as of now handling SPLs and giving licenses, those that have postponed usage, and states that are not individuals yet.

Further, as per the Center for Connected Health Policy (CCHP), there are nine state clinical or osteopathic sheets that issue uncommon licenses or testaments for telehealth that permit out-of-state suppliers to convey services using telemedicine in a state where they are not found or permit suppliers to convey telehealth services if certain criteria are met. Those states are:

- Alabama
- Louisiana
- Maine
- Minnesota
- New Mexico
- Ohio
- Oregon
- Tennessee (osteopathic board as it were)
- Texas

Telehealth Reimbursement

Another zone to know about with regards to telehealth is reimbursement. While each of the 50 states and the District of Columbia give repayment to some type of live video in the Medicaid expense for-administration model, just 21 have some type of repayment for remote patient checking in their Medicaid programs. Remote patient checking is characterized as the utilization of telehealth advancements to gather clinical information from patients in a single area and electronically transmit that data to a healthcare supplier in an alternate area. The states that offer RPM reimbursement are:

- Alabama
- Alaska
- Arizona
- Colorado
- Illinois
- Indiana
- Kansas
- Louisiana
- Maine
- Maryland
- Minnesota
- Mississippi
- Missouri
- Nebraska
- Oregon
- South Carolina

- Texas
- Utah
- Vermont
- Virginia
- Washington

Furthermore, just 11 state Medicaid programs incorporate repayment for store-and-forward services, which take into account the electronic transmission of clinical data, for example, computerized pictures and pre-recorded recordings:

- Alaska
- Arizona
- Connecticut
- California
- Georgia
- Maryland
- Minnesota
- New Mexico
- Nevada
- Virginia
- Washington

Informed Consent

At last, there are 38 states, including the District of Columbia, that have an educated assent necessity in their authoritative code, Medicaid strategies, or rules. Educated assent implies the patient comprehend the realities and risks associated with utilizing telehealth services.

Those states are:

- Alabama
- Arizona
- Arkansas
- California
- Colorado
- Connecticut
- Delaware
- Georgia
- Idaho
- Indiana
- Kansas
- Kentucky
- Louisiana
- Maine
- Maryland
- Michigan
- Minnesota (for alcohol and abuse programs)
- Mississippi
- Missouri
- Nebraska
- New Hampshire
- New Jersey
- New Mexico

- New York
- Ohio
- Oklahoma
- Oregon (for physical therapy and community treatment)
- Pennsylvania
- Rhode Island
- South Carolina
- Tennessee
- Texas
- Vermont
- Virginia
- Washington
- West Virginia
- Wisconsin
- Wyoming

17 Best Telemedicine Companies

It tends to be hard to make time to see your doctor. Between occupied schedule and restricted arrangement accessibility, remaining sound can prompt additional pressure. Telemedicine permits you to talk about non-emergency medical issues with a specialist by telephone or online during a period that is helpful for you.

Here are 17 of the best telemedicine organizations.

1. **CareClix**

CareClix was established in 2010. They work with board-affirmed practicing doctors to give a wide scope of telehealth and telemedicine benefits far and wide. A portion of the services they spread include:

- home care
- irresistible sicknesses
- pediatrics
- essential care
- urgent care

The organization additionally propelled a creative program for schools in Maryland. Utilizing Skype, off-site specialists can analyze grade school students, for example, those grumbling of an irritated throat, without the students leaving school grounds.

2. ConsultADoctor

If you have a non-emergency medical question, ConsultADoctor can help associate you with specialists by telephone and on the web. The organization spends significant time in offering essential clinical services that don't require visits face to face. If fundamental, specialists can likewise arrange tests and compose solutions that you can fill anyplace in the United States.

3. Teladoc

Teladoc was one of the first telehealth suppliers in the United States. They have kept up an exceptionally positive rating among doctors and patients. Ninety-two percent of Teladoc individuals have revealed that the conferences settled their medical questions. Teladoc additionally guarantees a normal callback time of a short ways from the minute an individual searches out a telephone or online video consultation.

Charges fluctuate contingent upon your arrangement. If you have an adaptable spending or wellbeing spending account, you might have the option to utilize it to cover benefits through Teladoc.

Teledoc can be utilized for a wide scope of medical issues, including:

- pediatric services
- non-emergency medical issues
- dermatological conditions
- psychological well-being discussions for issues, for example, depression and addiction
- sexual wellbeing consultations

Teladoc doctors can likewise compose medicines or break down your lab results.

4. MeMD

Making a record on MeMD is basic. When your record is set up, you can talk with a medical caretaker specialist or doctor legitimately through your computer's webcam.

You can talk about numerous side effects or conditions during a single consultation without expecting to pay an extra expense, gave your medicinal services supplier feels good examining a subsequent issue. Lab tests can't be requested through MeMD, yet healthcare suppliers can address inquiries concerning a current lab report.

5. iCliniq

The site iCliniq gives an assortment of services. You can submit composed inquiries or solicitation, a telephone counsel, or online video.

If you present a composed inquiry, one of the over 1,000 specialists speaking to around 80 distinct strengths will answer on the site. You can likewise get to filed questions and replies.

If you have to talk with a specialist, telephone, or online video counsels are accessible depending on the specialist's schedule. The organization additionally works as a "virtual hospital" for human services experts and clinical focuses.

Counsels are accessible in these areas:
- psychiatry
- oncology
- obstetrics and gynecology
- dentistry

- sexology
- dermatology
- general medication

6. American Well

Two siblings who are the two specialists established American Well. They needed to make basic health care progressively reasonable and dispense with obstructions, for example, separation, versatility, and time. Notwithstanding the site, American Well's mobile application, accessible on iPhone and Android, can likewise associate you with a specialist.

When utilizing the service, you'll be coordinated with specialists in your state. Notwithstanding broad medication questions, American Well likewise has emotional well-being advisors and nutritionists accessible for discussion. The organization is consistently developing its system of specialists.

7. MDlive

MDlive was established in 2009. They're persistently developing their associations with the healthcare system over the United States.

Board-affirmed doctors and other human services experts are accessible by telephone or online video 24 hours per day. They can help answer your inquiries regarding non-emergency medical conditions, for example,

- sensitivities
- urinary tract infections (UTIs)
- headaches
- rashes
- fever

Mental health professionals are, likewise accessible.

8. MDAligne

MDAligne has given more than 1 million on the web and phone conferences since 2004. They help individuals with a wide scope of wellbeing and health concerns.

MDAligne separates itself from some other telemedicine organizations by banding together with labs and imaging organizations. They additionally offer wellbeing enhancements and products for weight loss.

9. StatDoctors

StatDoctors has been around since 2009. They brag short hold up times to hear once again from specialists. The hold-up time is around six minutes. An across the country system of specialists is accessible 24 hours every day for telephone consultations or online video assessments.

10. Doctors on Demand

One thing that separates Doctor on Demand from its rivals is that it permits individuals to add a specialist to their "top choices." If that specialist is accessible, you can get back to them straightforwardly to make future arrangements.

Doctor on Demand likewise offers new mothers online help from board-certified location advisors.

11. Specialists On Call

Specialists on Call offer their types of assistance to emergency clinics and doctor practices rather than individual customers. The organization is planned as a counseling practice for clinical offices around the country.

If a hospital needs a stroke specialist, for instance, an on the web or telephone counsel is organized with one of the Specialists on Call's primary care physicians.

12. LiveHealth Online

LiveHealth Online lets individuals select the specialists they talk with using two-way video conferencing. When you join, you can see who's accessible in your state and afterward demand a consultation. You ought to be associated with the specialist you include picked inside a couple of moments.

Doctors are accessible 24 hours every day, seven days per week. LiveHealth Online's site additionally includes wellbeing tips.

13. Virtuwell

Virtuwell handles the diagnostic part of telemedicine by requesting that you depict your symptoms in an online meeting. If side effects and conditions sound like something Virtuwell can treat, a medical caretaker expert will get the report. They would then be able to take a gander at an obvious side effect, if essential, and make a treatment plan.

Conditions qualified for virtual consultations include:

- colds and flus
- acne
- birth control
- skin conditions
- certain sexually transmitted ailments
- sensitivities

Other fundamental non-emergency medical issues

14. Ringadoc

Ringadoc spends significant time in supporting different doctors by dealing with their twilight calls. At the point when you call, your condition will be triaged, and key data will be furnished to the specialists contracting with Ringadoc. The thought is that solitary dire calls are sent nightfall.

15. PlushCare

Notwithstanding coordinating you with a doctor for online video talks or calls, PlushCare likewise offers back to the community. With each meeting, PlushCare gives assets or services to help California kids get vaccinations or exams.

PlushCare is now accessible in eight states.

16. HealthTap

HealthTap cases to have 72,000 specialists around the globe prepared to respond to your wellbeing questions. Specialists are accessible for video visits or basically to answer instant messages. Their portable application, HealthTap, accessible on iPhone and Android, additionally gives wellbeing news.

17. HealthExpress

HealthExpress assists individuals in Oregon and Washington with non-emergency healthcare consultation. Consultations are accessible through telephone or two-way video conferencing.

Not at all like numerous telemedicine organizations, HealthExpress isn't open 24 hours. Doctors and nurse practitioners are accessible from 8 a.m. to 8 p.m. during the week and from 9 a.m. to 5 p.m. on ends of the week. You can go online and pick a medical professional to support you.

Accommodation and Affordability

Telemedicine makes it simpler than at any other time to get medical treatment. It's likewise a reasonable alternative for individuals without insurance.

Chapter 6

Types of Telemedicine

Telemedicine alludes to the delivery of clinical services a way off. The act of telemedicine, to a great extent, separates into three kinds of solutions, store-and-forward, remote patient monitoring, and real-time encounters.

Store-and-Forward Telemedicine

Store-and-forward telemedicine is likewise called "asynchronous telemedicine." It is a technique by which healthcare suppliers share understanding clinical data like lab reports, imaging studies, recordings, and different records with a doctor, radiologist, or master at another area. It isn't normal for email, yet it is finished utilizing an answer that has inherent, complex security highlights to guarantee patient confidentiality.

Store-and-forward telemedicine is a productive path for patients, essential consideration suppliers, and authorities to team up because they would all be able to review the data when it is helpful for them. The methodology gives patients access to a care group that can be contained by suppliers in various areas, even across significant distances and in various time zones.

Store-and-forward is especially well known for judgments and treatment with specific strengths, including dermatology, ophthalmology, and radiology.

Remote Patient Monitoring

Remote patient observation, or "telemonitoring," is a technique that permits healthcare experts to follow a patient's essential signs and exercises a good way off. This sort of observation is frequently utilized for the services of high-chance patients, similar to those with heart conditions and individuals who have as of late been released from the emergency clinic. Remote monitoring is likewise amazingly helpful for the treatment of various interminable conditions. It very well may be utilized by diabetics, for instance, to follow their glucose levels and send the information to their primary care physician. Older patients at home or in helped living offices can be advantageous and cheaply observed.

Real-time telemedicine

At the point when you consider telemedicine, it is likely continuous video visits that rings a bell. During an ongoing telemedicine experience, patients and suppliers use video conferencing programming to hear and see one another. While different kinds of telemedicine are utilized to improve conventional in-person visits, constant telemedicine can be utilized instead of an outing to the specialist's office in specific circumstances. It is famous for essential care, critical consideration, follow-up visits, and the administration of drugs and incessant disease.

Note that the consumer video correspondence applications that we use to interface with companions and associates, as Facetime and Skype, are not fitting for telemedicine. Telehealth experiences ought to be directed utilizing innovation that has been intended to secure patient security and meet the severe patient assurances required by the Health Insurance Portability and Accountability Act (HIPAA).

Each kind of telemedicine gives suppliers another approach to convey successful, productive consideration to patients. They extend access for patients and give a progressively advantageous approach to get the consideration they need.

9 MYTHS OF TELEMEDICINE

As a doctor with 20 years of involvement with an emergency room, I know the importance of "overpowered." It's anything but difficult to feel like you're stuck between a rock and a hard place when you're confronting an endless stream of patients with medical problems little and huge.

Numerous doctors feel a similar frenzy when they look at the wellbeing technology alternatives that are accessible today. With each kind of program, application, and gadget a couple of snaps away, it's hard not to be distrustful when given another bit of tech.

I accept that it is the reason numerous doctors never really think about telemedicine. For some explanation, specialists let our distrustful sides outwit us since we think a great deal of the "following enormous things" is only a prevailing fashion.

In any case, telemedicine isn't going anyplace. It is anything but a trend. I ensure telemedicine will have a colossal job later on for medication - to a great extent, since it carries a huge amount of advantages to the two specialists and patients.

I've conversed with numerous specialists about telemedicine as I'm clarifying what eVisit does. A larger part of the time, doctors who state they're not intrigued simply don't have a lot of involvement in telemedicine and don't completely see how it very well may be utilized to profit their training. Their contentions against telemedicine are founded on normal legends - they don't hold up when I clarify the realities.

When I clarify precisely what telemedicine resembles practically speaking and expose those legends, a larger part of specialists are prepared to come locally available - or are in any event open to considering telemedicine. So the test is teaching suppliers about that misinformation. What's valid about telemedicine and so forth?

As a doctor and as the prime supporter of eVisit, I'm fortunate to have a remarkable point of view: I've utilized telemedicine stages and taken part in building one. In case you're a doctor who's still reeling about utilizing telemedicine in your training, investigate these regular fantasies, and check whether you alter your perspective.

1. I have to do a physical test

A few specialists contend that an in-person test is important to give quality medical care. While an in-person test is significant in numerous situations, there are as yet a huge amount of conditions that don't require one. Simply think about all the conditions you've treated via telephone before. For some, minor dire conditions, knowing the patient's clinical history and the announced side effects is sufficient to analyze without a physical test. Moreover, telemedicine is truly significant for basic follow-up calls or post-operation registrations that, for the most part, don't require a physical test in any case.

2. Telemedicine technology is excessively overpowering

Utilizing innovation in your training can be unpleasant, confounding, and even terrifying. I get this. Be that as it may, embracing innovation is inescapable, and it doesn't need to be outlandish. Search for telemedicine arrangements that were worked with doctor input - they're bound to be effortlessly adjusted to your work process. At the point when you're looking, additionally, assess how easy to understand the stage is, how much equipment or set-up you'll require, and what the merchant accommodates preparing. Search for a telemedicine stage that addresses your issues, and centers on making the supplier experience as simple as could be expected under the circumstances. There are telemedicine suppliers that meet every one of these criteria and can offer you stages that aren't significantly more entangled than Skype or Facetime.

3. I won't be made up for my time

Telemedicine raises your pay. Numerous specialists are amazed to hear this since they're centered around the repayment angle. However, think about this - what amount of time have you spent on uncompensated twilight calls? On medicine tops off? Transforming these utilization cases into telemedicine visits can recover remuneration. Numerous telemedicine visits are additionally now reimbursable through Medicare, Medicaid, and private payers - particularly the same number of states currently have telemedicine equality laws.

Besides, we've discovered that patients are regularly ready to pay a level charge only for the accommodation of doing a telemedicine visit.

4. It won't work with my EMR

The facts demonstrate that some telemedicine stages don't coordinate with an EMR. Be that as it may, many do offer combinations, or produce a visit record that can be sent out into your EMR.

5. It will be excessively expensive

While it depends on what sort of telemedicine program you need to assemble, telemedicine doesn't need to be costly. In case you're simply keen on offering patients an approach to do virtual visits for basic registration, incessant consideration the board, lab results conversations, your telemedicine arrangement doesn't have to include significantly more than access to a computer, webcam, and amplifier, alongside the proper web or versatile application. Without the additional gear needs, programming establishment and set-up, and included instructional courses - telemedicine can be a reasonable alternative in any event for little practices.

It's likewise critical to take note of that telemedicine can help your training income, and conveys an incredible ROI.

6. My patients won't use it

This comes as an amazement to certain doctors: patients love telemedicine. As per a 2015 review by Software Advice, just 16% of patients would like to look for care at a crisis room if they additionally had the alternative of telemedicine. Perhaps that is because 97% of patients are disappointed by specialist's office to hold up times, however, perhaps they simply love the comfort of being treated with no drive and no bother.

7. It will build the risk of malpractice

Telemedicine can diminish your danger of misbehavior by including another opportunity for documentation of treatment. It additionally encourages subsequent meet-ups and permits you to accomplish progressively visit registration to ensure patients are remaining on target and clinging to treatment. Regardless of whether you're an orthopedic specialist with a full calendar of post-operation arrangements, or an attendant specialist monitoring a patient with an infection, telemedicine gives you more purposes of contact.

8. It's not secure

Dissimilar to Skype, and other video talk advancements, telemedicine platforms are HIPAA consistent and frequently designed with military-grade security. In case you're at all worried about security hazards, simply ask the telemedicine supplier how they've manufactured their foundation to guarantee 100% security and consistency with HIPAA.

9. It just won't work for me

Like I said previously, specialists are wary essentially - credit it to being unreasonably brilliant to our benefit. In any case, I can let you know as a matter of the fact that I've seen specialists from varying backgrounds (even the individuals who guarantee they aren't "well informed") give shot telemedicine and bedazzled with the outcomes. Everything necessary is the readiness to find out more and give it a shot in your training.

Ways Telehealth Leads to Higher Patient Satisfaction Levels

"Patient-centered care" is probably the most blazing trendy expression in healthcare at present.

Surely, almost all human services change endeavors — including the Affordable Care Act — look to join unique wellbeing frameworks and suppliers under the shared objective of guaranteeing that every individual patient gets the correct treatment from the correct professional at the perfect time. Furthermore, as a rule, "ideal time" signifies "right this moment."

Generally, however, giving patients on-request healthcare was everything except inconceivable; even crisis room visits regularly require a holding up period among appearance and assessment. With the approach of telehealth, however, patients have the intensity of on-request medicinal services readily available — and that is extraordinary news for suppliers hoping to improve understanding fulfillment.

Here's the reason:

1) It empowers quicker care delivery— and along these lines, better results.

With numerous conditions, the quicker the patient gets treatment, the better the potential consequences of that treatment. As such, when patients sit tight for treatment — either because they would prefer not to experience the issue of setting up an arrangement or they can't jump on the supplier's calendar quickly — their infirmities regularly decline, which makes it significantly harder for the specialist to reestablish them to full wellbeing.

At the point when patients look for treatment using telehealth, then again, there are far fewer boundaries to provoke care conveyance — which implies patients can jump on the way to recuperation before their conditions deteriorate. That, thus, prompts better patient results — and higher patient fulfillment levels.

2) It's simpler in the patient pocketbook.

Research has demonstrated that telehealth services are less expensive than human services conveyed in a traditional setting—at the individual visit level, yet also as far as downstream cost investment funds. As announced here, "the evaluated cost distinction between a telehealth visit and a comparing office-based visit is generally $40, after altering for what occurs after the visit."

To repeat my point from number one above, brief consideration conveyance keeps patients' conditions from declining, which by and large enable those patients to maintain a strategic distance from the requirement for progressively complex — and increasingly costly — treatment.

Also, as a rule, the fewer cash patients need to dish out for healthcare benefits, the more joyful those patients are.

3) It causes patients to feel like they are the need.

Nobody likes to feel disregarded or ignored. What's more, when a patient is wiped out or in torment — and the individual in question is advised to hold on in the lounge area until a specialist is accessible — it's simple for that patient to feel like the person in question doesn't make a difference. To the extent, tolerant fulfillment goes, that is an intense gap for any supplier to uncover oneself from underneath — paying little heed to how outstanding their treatment is.

Telemedicine, then again, permits patients to sidestep negative lounge area encounters — which implies they go into their patient-specialist cooperations with a lot higher benchmark level of fulfillment.

4) It permits suppliers to see more patients.

In physical clinical workplaces, a supplier's capacity to plan an arrangement for the patient's ideal date and time is dependent upon treatment room accessibility. There are just such a large number of rooms in the structure — which implies there's a predetermined number of arrangement openings on the schedule.

Indeed, as indicated by an investigation referred to right now, normal time new patients need to stand by to see a specialist in 15 metropolitan areas the nation over is 18 days. Telehealth takes out those planning imperatives, opening up suppliers to see more patients — and make increasingly fulfilled clients.

The present customers — including healthcare customers — have exclusive standards. Also, for occupied medicinal services suppliers with restricted assets, meeting those desires can be intense.

Yet, in the present change driven healthcare condition, the significance of patient fulfillment will just keep on developing — which implies suppliers can't manage the cost of not searching for creative approaches to keep their patients fulfilled.

Chapter 7

Building a Telehealth Program: Where Do I Start?

Urgency, as it identifies with healthcare, is the same old thing. Who hasn't griped about sitting in minimal more than a paper sheet for what feels like hours just to experience a normal yearly physical? Individuals need to realize that they are sound, and they would prefer not to need to hang tight for the non-literal green light before coming back to everyday life. On-request care has been a looked for after assistance for quite a long time paying little heed to what you experience the ill effects of strep throat, a messed up wrist or something incessant like Congestive Heart Failure.

Right now, of keen innovation and expanded correspondence and contact, we as patients anticipate every minute of everyday access to all things - and human services are no exemption. How is this cultivated, however, and how would we train clinical staff in an ever-developing business sector that in the not so distant past existed uniquely in explicit specialties of the populace? Telehealth offers the mind-blowing potential to convey quicker, more financially savvy care that by the day's end is likewise better for the patient. Be that as it may, this is no simple task.

Discover Your Flag-Bearers

It's nothing unexpected that we are best at things we are enthusiastic about. There are special cases to this, yet as a rule, suppliers give the best consideration when they love what they do. Human services are specific, and telehealth is only one part of the many-furnished monster we know as the clinical field. Nevertheless, medical caretakers and doctors in every aspect of healthcare ought to be excited for what they do and propelled to serve their patients. So what happens when suppliers are emotionless about their telehealth benefits or are making an insincere effort since it's their activity?

While the advantages of telehealth are various, there is an opposite potential for diminished nature of patient consideration and separate from patients with an enormous and to some degree undedicated group. Each patient presents a chance to change and improve a real existence through legitimate consideration, social association, and friendship. Without such an attitude, in any case, both the patient and supplier are in danger for the poor by and large consideration and general disappointment with the telehealth program.

It is imperative to perceive the energetic people who will support your telehealth program and try to improve the personal satisfaction for each enlisted quiet. By the day's end, healthcare isn't and shouldn't be "only work," yet rather a guarantee of helping other people. Telehealth can be requesting and, on occasion, very testing. However, having the correct mentality has a significant effect. No patient needs to experience an activity if their specialist is contemplating an up and coming golf trip, or about the profession in law she ought to have sought after. The equivalent is valid for a telehealth program and its individuals. It is basic to locate your committed and empathetic group, whose people tune in to, comprehend, and look to improve the requirements of their patients.

Support Hand-Raising

One of the numerous characteristics that makes somebody a good leader is their ability to instruct and to educate by model. Without the capacity to impart one's vision to a group and plan on the best way to best accomplish certain objectives, the outcomes you're searching for likely won't work out as expected. In any case, similarly that speaking with and encouraging others adequately prompts a solid inner group, we should likewise concentrate on the possibility that posing inquiries can frequently be more significant than noting them.

Many feel that leaders should hold all the appropriate responses; in any case, the inquiries being posed are what genuinely drive the beneficial discussion. As Jeff Boss puts it, "questions sparkle interest, interest makes thoughts and [good] thoughts lead to development."

Healthcare associations today face unmatched difficulties to improve quality, increment gets to, streamline effectiveness, and cut expenses. Thus the requirement for development becomes in like manner to convey precaution and progressively customized care.

Enter the telehealth stage left.

telehealth nursing the objective toward the day's end is to give unrivaled and progressively proactive consideration at a small amount of the expense with innovation, at that point we should initially start by posing the inquiry, "where do we start?" such huge numbers of individuals, particularly in human services, are reluctant to approach even straightforward inquiries because of a paranoid fear of appearing to be inept. For some, there is a worry that posing inquiries will open ways to risk, disappointment, and shame, when unexpectedly, the request goes about as a solid helper much of the time.

Questions ought to be utilized to leverage problem solving and fuel discussion, and its an obvious fact that we have a ton of issues to understand with regards to the present condition of medicinal services in the United States and at the worldwide level. Direct inquiries inside your group to start enthusiasm and creativity, challenge colleagues to think past the self-evident, and banter over prescribed procedures. IDEO, known for its human-focused structure, utilizes the "In what capacity may we?" approach in three different ways:

1. "How" suggests that the current issue can in actuality be understood

2. "Might" recommends that beyond what one technique can exist when taking care of the issue

3. "We" shows that the arrangement can be found by filling in as a group. As opposed to fear questions, grasp them.

Challenge the Status Quo

Patients experiencing interminable conditions advantage essentially from protection measures planned for diminishing the seriousness and development of their analyses. For quite a while, telehealth has been utilized to solely target ceaseless consideration patients most in danger for medical clinic readmission. Telehealth permits suppliers to hand over the directing wheel of their patients' consideration the board to the patients themselves by offering instruments that upgrade commitment, instruction, and correspondence.

These very tools make it simpler for patients and doctors to remain associated and engage patients to get more beneficial, tending to two of the fundamental factors that add to avoidable ER visits and hospital readmissions. Everybody wins, correct? Be that as it may, shouldn't something be said about patients who don't experience the ill effects of ceaseless conditions? Shouldn't something is said about patients determined to have emotional wellness or conduct wellbeing issue, among others?

Supplier deficiencies and expanding quantities of mental and social wellbeing patients are making gaps in the delivery of care to these populaces; however, telehealth might be the answer for giving auspicious and practical consideration for all patients paying little heed to find. Lately, the interest for mental and conduct wellbeing administrations have had a considerable and expensive effect on healthcare organizations across the nation, particularly in Emergency Departments.

In 2013 alone, treatment for mental health disorders cost the country $201 billion, more than that spent to treat coronary illness or malignant growth. However, contemplates show that upwards of 44 million Americans experience a type of conduct wellbeing emergency every year. Still, then 60 percent of those influenced don't look for treatment at all on account of an absence of access or assets.

There is a lot of calculated work required to dispatch such projects, yet why not use telehealth to serve patients looking for help in the ED because of poor access to conduct and emotional wellness offices? Telehealth stands to beat obstructions by offering human services access to patients from the solace of their homes and workplaces.

Cautious, snappy, and reasonable, telemental and telebehavioral wellbeing administrations remain to offer looked for after consideration any place and at whatever point required. Not, at this point, only a trendy expression, telehealth is a practical treatment alternative for developing patient populaces, which no longer should be restricted to ceaseless care alone.

Chapter 8

How Much Does It Cost to Develop a Telemedicine App Like Doctor on Demand?

Three minutes. That is the normal time a patient wait to connect with a specialist utilizing Doctor on Demand. No big surprise, this application has caused a stir and now has more than a million enlisted clients. The application has become so well known that numerous centers and private business visionaries are currently pondering, creating comparative applications for themselves. So what does it take to begin a telemedicine application improvement?

What is Doctor on Demand?

Doctor on Demand empowers fast video consultations with experts. The application offers interviews every minute of every day and runs on cell phones, tablets, and computers. During a video meeting with a specialist, a patient offers side effects, gets a full conference, gets an analysis, and is given a solution or, now and again, a rundown of lab tests they should run. Among the most widely recognized conditions that patients treat utilizing the application are cold and flu, rashes, urinary tract contaminations, and allergies.

As should be obvious, everything is basic. Simplicity is one of the fundamental reasons why patients like the application to such an extent. Here are the most recent numbers that mirror its prevalence and achievement.

Why are telemedicine applications so popular?

The motivation behind why telemedicine applications have immense potential is that they offer points of interest for the two patients and specialists. This takes care of the chicken and egg issue.

Advantages that pull in patients

- **Comfort.** Making arrangements ahead of time, heading to a facility, and holding up in a long queue isn't the most advantageous approach to get a specialist's help. 74 percent of patients lean toward simple access to medicinal services benefits over the face to face communications with suppliers. This number is higher in the country and remote zones. In the US, for every 100,000 rustic patients, there are just 43 authorities accessible.
- **Spare time and get results quicker**. Patients spare time on counsels as well as can begin treatment straight away, directly after

the video call closes. This diminishes treatment time and gives quick outcomes.
- **Medical record versatility**. Indeed, even in the advanced world, it's as yet hard to gain admittance to your electronic clinical records, also another person's information. A telemedicine application permits patients to see their clinical records and send them to relatives and specialists.

Advantages that pull in doctors

- **Adaptability**. As indicated by Doctor on Demand, 20 percent of specialists and doctors work 60-to 80-hour weeks, and 15 percent concede they have discouragement that adversely impacts their productivity. Also, 15 percent of respondents who report sadness dread that their downturn could make them make blunders that they wouldn't customarily make. Working using a telemedicine application, specialists can pick their schedule.
- **Less regulatory work**. A lot of a doctor's workday is spent on managerial assignments and administrative work. Subsequently, specialists analyze fewer patients and need to remain after work to round out all the desk work. A telemedicine application limits desk work and computerizes a lot of tasks.

- **More patients and more income**. Less desk work implies more patients. What's more, more patients implies more income.

Highlights of a telemedicine application

If you need to begin your telemedicine application improvement, you need a rundown of must-have highlights. The Doctor on Demand stage has various interfaces, with various capabilities, for specialists and patients.

Highlights for patients

Profiles

To make a profile, a patient enters their name, address, sex, age, medical history, and other essential information required to begin the treatment procedure.

Book an arrangement

A client can see a rundown of specialists, see their profiles, and book a meeting with the specialist they pick. This component is one of the most pivotal because it gives patients data about a specialist's accessibility and lets them book a period that is reasonable for them.

Video conferencing

Patients utilize this element when they need a specialist to look at them. Doctors perform starting perceptions through video talk, which is the reason video quality is so significant. Appropriate analysis and precise treatment rely upon a smooth association and clear picture.

Voice-only calls

About psychological problems, a few people would prefer not to show their countenances and like to communicate incognito. For these reasons, the application offers a voice-just call highlight. It gives a protected channel to individuals who feel humiliated to discuss their issues to get qualified help.

Cloud-based e-record storage

When patients have made their records, they get e-Medical record stockpiling that contains all their data, including medical data and correspondence history. If important, these records can be imparted to another master, a life partner, or another relative.

Medication tracker

The application stores all medicines that a specialist composes and sends notifications to remind patients to take their medication.

Geolocation

As indicated by US clinical guidelines, a telemedicine application must associate patients with doctors authorized inside the express the patients are truly situated in. For these reasons, the Doctor on Demand application utilizes Google Maps to decide a client's area. Clients can likewise observe a guide to discover the closest drug store to get their solutions.

Built-in chat

A patient can utilize the safe implicit talk to contact a specialist with any dire inquiry, to get a subsequent conference, or if they have any inquiries concerning endorsed meds.

Payment gateway

Doctor on Demand permits patients to pay by credit or platinum card. It acknowledges all significant charge cards: Visa, Mastercard, American Express, and Discover. Patients may likewise pay utilizing HSA or FSA platinum cards as long as they have a Visa or Mastercard logo.

Rating and reviews

After an interview or after recuperation, a client can rate the specialist and leave a survey. This element enables new patients to settle on better decisions while searching for doctors.

Highlights for doctors
Profiles

A specialist needs to give their name, address, photograph, specialization, and accessibility. They can likewise give information about their experience and training.

Scheduling

Specialists can make changes to their schedules, depending on their accessibility.

Manage appointments

Doctors can see their full list of arrangements and acknowledge or dismiss them.

Live video calls

Video calls help specialists to look at patients all the more definitely. A specialist can request that a patient show their skin or throat, for example, to see a sore very close and make a conclusion.

Specialists can likewise utilize voice-only calls and built-in chat options to speak with patients.

Electronic medical records
Specialists approach clinical records of every one of their patients whenever they need it.

Digital prescriptions

Doctor on Demand permits specialists to recommend medication directly in the application. Patients can utilize these solutions to purchase medication or to get other wellbeing administrations at clinical foundations.

The reality: The component records are quite comparative for the two interfaces. Simultaneously, patients and specialists approach just those highlights they need the most. For instance, for patients, it's fundamental to approach individual profiles so they can follow their arrangements and results (like treatment plans and solutions). The most significant highlights for specialists are associated with their timetables. That is the reason they can screen and oversee plans directly from their profiles.

How telemedicine applications bring in cash

Doctor on Demand doesn't have a membership expense. It doesn't offer any exceptional records either. All highlights are accessible from the beginning. So how can it bring in cash? The application charges a 25 percent expense to patients each time they pay for a meeting. The expense for a little while relies upon the length and on the specialist:

- Medical doctor: $75 for a 15-minute discussion
- Therapist: $79 for a 25-minute conference, $119 for a 50-minute discussion
- Specialist: $229 for a 45-minute beginning discussion, $99 for a 15-minute follow-up visit

Notwithstanding, an exchange expense isn't the main route Doctor on Demand brings in the cash. It additionally gives its product as a help, offering its product to other clinical foundations. Doctor on Demand charges these SaaS clients for each supplier expense. Organizations that utilization Doctor on Demand programming pay for every worker consistently. This expense is about $1 per individual every month, so if an organization has 100,000 workers, it would cost about $1.2 million consistently.

Here are some different ways to deal with adapting your telemedicine application:

- Yearly participation for patients. The Arizona Telemedicine Program utilizes this adaptation procedure. Its clients pay a yearly expense and a charge for each assistance they get.
- Month to month expense for specialists and patients. This methodology requires the two patients and specialists to pay an expense each month to utilize the product. Myca

Nutrition utilizes this methodology and establishments its framework to different nations.
- Franchising. If your neighborhood advertise is packed, why not go to another market? This is actually what SkyHealth did. SkyHealth is a nongovernmental association situated in the United States. The organization offers its establishment to wellbeing associations for just $3,000.
- A per-minute charge. Right now, tolerant pays for each moment of a counsel with authority. The Tele Doctoral program, possessed by the Norwegian Telenor Group, charges $US0.08 every moment for a telephone discussion with a specialist.

Difficulties of building up a telemedicine application

Building a telemedicine application, similar to any clinical application, includes certain difficulties, including security and legitimate consistency. Here's a short outline of what you should remember when you start your telemedicine application improvement:

#1. Security concerns

Private wellbeing data is delicate. Telemedicine applications gather and store data and, normally, this makes clients wonder if their wellbeing information is in a protected spot and who approaches it.

Solution. To secure your clients, you should actualize different factor validation, recognizable biometric proof (like the face or fingerprint ID), and information encryption. These measures improve the security of your application and shield it from information ruptures.

#2. Absence of trust

Another worry is associated with specialists' capabilities. Patients need to be certain that they're speaking with a certified proficient, not with a fresh university graduate.

Solution. Tributes from patients and a straightforward rating framework can convince your clients. You can likewise permit specialists to give to their web-based life profiles so patients can become more acquainted with their doctors from another, progressively close to the home side.

#3. Consistency with healthcare legislation

Various nations have their demonstrations and laws that direct the assortment, preparing, stockpiling, and sharing of individual wellbeing data. In the USA, it's HIPAA. In Canada, it's PIPEDA. European Union nations follow the Data Protection Directive 1995/46/EC and the e-Privacy Directive 2002/58/EC. Your telemedicine application needs to agree to the laws in the nation where it works.

Solution. Focus on the laws managing clinical information handling in the nation your application will work in. Pick an advancement organization that has experience creating HIPAA or PIPEDA consistent frameworks to be certain that the item you create with be agreeable and won't bring about any lawful issues later on.

Chapter 9

Employment

On account of innovation, work-life balance and remote working are feasible for those in the medical industry. Remote jobs are readily available for medical workers in different areas, allowing them to give clinical help from the comfort of their own home. Read on to study adaptable occupations in telemedicine.

What Are Telemedicine and Telehealth Jobs?

Concurring an ongoing Forbes article, "Telemedicine, or 'telehealth,' is the arrangement of remote access to a doctor using telephone or videoconference to address a health care issue." Telemedicine can offer quicker support to patients, removes travel, allows patient's access to specialists found several miles away and can relieve in-office staffing issues. Typical duties include virtually consulting, talking with patients, surveying quiet records, giving treatment choices, and then some.

Telemedicine opportunities can give prepared experts either all-day work or essentially side work to occupy in their available time.

Basic Jobs and Who's Hiring

Flexible jobs in telemedicine run the gamut. You'll discover remote positions in almost every industry, for example, pharmaceutical, nursing, clinical, pediatric, nutrition, and mental health. Regular occupation titles are like what you'd find for in-office positions: specialist, nurture, clinical coder, nutritionist, clinical executive, drug specialist, and so on. Organizations enlisting for employments in telemedicine incorporate Humana, IDEXX Laboratories, Aetna, UnitedHealth Group, and SpecialtyCare.

In case you're in the market for a remote telehealth work, here's testing of 12 jobs hiring now.

1. Internal Medicine Consultant II

2. Clinician

3. Neuromonitoring Physician

4. Internal Medicine Consultant II

5. Radiologist II

6. Oncology Abstractor

7. Obstetrics – Gynecology Medical Review Physician

8. Telehealth Nurse

9. Board-Certified Physician

10. Pharmacist – Clinical Advisor

11. Nurse Medical Management

12. Medical Director

Telehealth Models for Promoting Workforce Recruitment and Retention

In rural communities that are facing deficiencies of doctors and physicians, telehealth can be utilized as an instrument to advance workforce recruitment. For instance, telehealth models can allow rural communities to actualize alternative staffing models. Numerous telehealth programs allow advanced practice clinicians, experts, and other healthcare workers to practice at the highest point of their permit while accepting remote supervision from a doctor or other clinician. Contingent upon the telehealth model, managing doctors, may watch a live video feed, survey quiet records, or speak with rustic staff using phone.

Also, younger providers who have been prepared in the utilization of health information technologies might be more urged to rehearse in a rural facility that has a telehealth foundation set up. Providers who are unwilling to move to country regions may also be willing to "work from home" on a section or full-time basis.

Telehealth can help retain rural healthcare workers by encouraging contact with different providers, decreasing feelings of isolation, and offering open doors for proceeding with medical education. Receiving additional support from different experts may enable rural providers to keep away from burnout. For instance, telehealth consultation services can help ease the remaining burden of rural providers who are relied upon to play out different capacities given workforce shortages. One investigation of rustic clinicians and hospital administrators found that telehealth helped enlist and hold family practice doctors by distributing the obligations of being available to come into work for emergency services.

Instances of Recruitment and Retention through Telehealth

• The North Dakota Telepharmacy Project (NDTP) has increased recruitment and retention of drug store benefits across country North Dakota. Preceding project usage, 26 country drug stores in the state had shut because of financial concerns, difficulty recruiting qualified pharmacists to rural areas, and other operational difficulties. NDTP causes address barriers to the workforce lack by allowing a drug store technician to apportion solutions under the supervision of a pharmacist through telehealth. The program has effectively made over 80 new jobs in rural North Dakota.

• The Humboldt General Hospital EMS Rescue service in rural Nevada utilizes telehealth to help train and recruit employees and volunteers. The rescue service partners with the Great Basin College Emergency Medical Services Program to give preparing to nearby Humboldt staff and volunteers through videoconferencing. Thus, Humboldt offers work experience situations to Great Basin students. Humboldt has effectively enlisted and procured Great Basin students after they finished their program.

• Acadia Hospital, some portion of the Eastern Maine Healthcare Systems, utilizes telehealth to give every minute of every day psychiatric consultations to medical providers at rural emergency departments. The telepsychiatry program has assisted with tending to long-standing difficulties in recruiting qualified behavioral health providers in rural Maine. Suppliers are all the more ready to join Acadia Hospital due to the chance to practice remotely. In addition to psychiatrists and psychiatric attendant experts who are situated in

Maine, the program additionally incorporates psychiatry staff from Massachusetts and Indiana.

Implementation Considerations

Projects trying to set up a claim to staff specialty services with technicians or advanced practice clinicians ought to know about state rules that control remote supervision by doctors. For instance, a few states don't allow advanced practice medical caretakers to get supervision through telehealth. Projects may need to talk with state sheets of medication, nursing, and drug store to guarantee they are in consistence with telehealth regulations. Furthermore, programs that recruit staff across state lines ought to know about challenges related to licensing and credentialing.

Country programs hoping to select recruit pharmacy technicians, dental assistants and hygienists, nurture assistants, and other healthcare workers with partner degrees may try to construct organizations with local community colleges. Rural programs can offer preparing experience to students and give data about telehealth applications. For instance, the pharmacy technician program at the North Dakota State College of Science incorporates Telepharmacy models in its curriculum.

Public Policy Implications

Public policies can inhibit the spread of tele-emergency and different kinds of telehealth. Barriers to execution incorporate Medicare strategies identified with payment and states of investment, state approaches including authorizing and credentialing guidelines, Medicaid installment and on-location staffing necessities, and private-segment payment policies. Conversely, other public policies, for example, shared payment programs, value-based buying, and regulatory policy changes explicitly intended to suit telehealth—can energize its utilization. This mixed approach condition can engender confusion yet additionally makes open doors for the expansion of telehealth.

For services delivered using tele-crisis, Medicare repays basic access clinics dependent on the expense of giving care, including charges paid to a tele-emergency hub. However, Medicare does, Medicare doesn't repay clinics for an initial purchase of tele-emergency equipment, and other private and open payers don't, for the most part, repay reimburse access emergency clinics on a cost basis.

Along these lines, under current strategies, the full expense of tele-emergency care can't go exclusively through reimbursement for services rendered. With tele-emergency, the absolute expense of care likely could be not as much as options including travel to another site to get care that could have been furnished locally with the contribution of clinicians at a center site. However, it is hard to confirm the cost reserve funds from decreased patient exchanges. With additional financial benefits to the basic access medical clinic and health system coming about because of more patient care (counting inpatient care following the intervention in the emergency room), absolute incomes may exceed costs regardless of underpayment for the telehealth service.

Since clinicians in tele-emergency center points serve multiple distant sites, cross-state clinician authorizing is another test to tele-emergency implementation. Efforts to address this issue incorporate the National Council of State Boards of Nursing's interstate medical nurse licensure compact, through which twenty-four states have consented to acknowledge another state's license for nurses

States have additionally investigated utilizing constrained licenses for telehealth and sped up consent to practice in one state for doctors authorized in another state. In 2006 the Office for the Advancement of Teleheath in the Health Resources and Services Administration made the Licensure Portability Grant Program to support state clinical sheets' efforts to wipe out hurdles coming about because of cross-state licenses issues.

A large number of our interviewees referenced the Emergency Medical Treatment and Active Labor Act (EMTALA) of 1986, which expects EDs to give balancing out treatment to patients, as a barrier to realizing the full advantages of tele-emergency implementation. Until the Centers for Medicare and Medicaid Services gave direction in 2013, rural hospital administrators we interviewed accepted that they were required to utilize an on-call staff if the need arises staff doctor to back up a doctor assistant or nurse practitioner in the ED, in any event, when prompt access to physician backup was available using tele-emergency.

The new regulatory guidance permits critical-access hospitals to meet all commitments under EMTALA and the Medicare states of investment with an on-location doctor right hand or attendant expert and a physician available using tele-emergency technology. Our interviewees proposed that this regulatory interpretation has facilitated the emergency call burden in rural areas, removing any other barrier regarding recruiting and retaining rural physicians.

Tele-Emergency's Role in Connected Health

Taken together, original research recommend that tele-emergency expands access to high-quality, incorporated, patient-centered care, and particularly in rural areas. Tele-crisis grows access to strength care in rural areas directly by adding assets to the care team. Tele-emergency's circuitous impacts are also significant. In rural hospitals, tele-crisis can increase both the help for local clinicians and community members' trust in their care. This procedure balances out the patient base and clinical assets on which rural hospitals depend for their proceeding with continuing viability.

Tele-emergency advances incorporation between critical-access hospitals and urban crisis clinicians and can improve care quality by giving providers in various areas access to different health care delivery assets. Planning care through tele-crisis shows patient-focused and gives patients the right care at the opportune time. Pre-established communication methodologies encourage crisis moves of patients to the proper setting quickly and effectively. The strategies also decline the number of pointless exchanges for patients who—using tele-emergency—can be securely treated in their community hospitals.

In a period of expanding rivalry for physicians and nurses, tele-emergency is a method for holding nearby fundamental providers. By giving backup backing to nurses in-country EDs, tele-emergency can circulate nursing assets productively over various rural settings. Tele-emergency encourages the enlistment and maintenance of physicians in rural areas, a considerable lot of whom fill in as family practitioners when not accepting brings in the ED. Subsequently, tele-crisis might be a way not exclusively to increase rural access to emergency care yet, also, to hold family specialists in rural areas.

Tele-emergency care connects clinicians in manners that extend the group of providers thinking about a patient during a period of emergency, improving clinical quality, and patients' trust in the treatment gave. Moreover, patients' ideal encounters with local care in a clinic ED makes a feeling that different services are also of top-notch since nearby providers are associated with extra ability varying. Patients are also prone to feel that they need not travel away from their local encouraging group of people for care. Telehealth builds up associations among clinicians and patients and distant providers, making the chance of integrated care inside regional delivery systems—either single associations or affiliations of independent providers.

Financial benefits accrue from diminished patient transfers and from considering at least costly setting. However, cost-based reimbursement may not take care of all expenses of care. As payment systems, for example, those dependent on total care value or shared reserve funds, advance to help cost-effective models of integrated care, telehealth will turn out to be all the more financially appealing for singular suppliers and health care systems.

Significance of Sustainability Planning for Telehealth Programs

To achieve sustainability, rural telehealth programs may need to show that the program has measurably affected the lives of individuals served by the program and the overall community. Evaluation activities can help show this incentive by following progress on process and outcome measures of telehealth programs.

Long-term sustainability also relies on the successful implementation and adoption of telehealth services. The Northeast Telehealth Resource Center's Roadmap for Planning Development of Clinical Telemedicine Services gives key considerations to coordinating maintainability procedures into program planning. For instance, country projects ought to evaluate their patient mix and protection status to decide how reimbursement policies will influence their maintainability plans.

Numerous telehealth programs additionally build up a field-tested strategy to plan for long-term sustainability. Key considerations for country networks creating business or sustainability plans include:

• Understanding the interest for telehealth in the network and the sorts of methodologies that will best address recognized issues

• Assessing the current work process and identifying what sorts of assets are expected to incorporate telehealth into training

• Identifying a victor to drive telehealth appropriation, address issues, and identify programs for proceeded with use

• Providing sufficient preparing and backing for staff to guarantee the ideal experience for staff and patients

- Budgeting for usage, support, and periodic upgrades of technology

- Marketing telehealth services to network individuals, suppliers, and different partners

- Understanding the regulatory environment to understand progressing costs for repayment, licensing, and credentialing

- Building organizations with payers to extend inclusion for telehealth services

The Telehealth Resource Centers give free specialized help to provincial networks trying to make manageability plans for telehealth programs.

Maintainability Strategies for Rural Telehealth Programs

There are several different strategies for sustaining telehealth programs that might be helpful for rural healthcare systems and providers. The Rural Community Health Toolkit also gives data about general Sustainability Strategies and Sustainability Strategies for Specific Issues. Extra data about funding for rural telehealth tasks and frameworks can be found in the Telehealth Use in Rural Healthcare topic guide.

Repayment for Telehealth Services

A few provincial telehealth programs depend on repayments from Medicare, Medicaid, and private back up plans to fund telehealth services.

Medicare requires the "beginning site" of telehealth, which refers to the area of the Medicare recipient at the time they get telehealth services, to be a district outside of a Metropolitan Statistical Area (MSA) or to be a provincial Health Professional Shortage Area (HPSA) situated in a rural census tract. The Health Resources and Services Administration's Medicare Telehealth Payment Eligibility Analyzer tool can assist networks with deciding their qualification for Medicare repayments. CMS gives direction to explain repayment arrangements for Medicare charge for-specialist co-ops. CMS additionally built up a booklet called Rural Providers and Suppliers Billing.

Medicaid and private payer reimbursement rates generally shift from state to state. The Center for Connected Health Policy screens current state laws and repayment approaches and reports on state telehealth laws and reimbursement practices.

When getting ready for long long-term sustainability, rural communities ought to know about the following considerations for reimbursements:

•   Parity laws at the government and state-level decide if telehealth visits are repaid at a similar rate as face to face visits. The American Telemedicine Association tracks equality laws for private protection inclusion of telehealth.

•   Payers may put various limitations on the starting site for telehealth services. Rural programs ought to survey in the case of beginning site limitations that will permit them to give telehealth benefits outside of healthcare settings, for example, in patients' homes or schools.

- Payers may also limit reimbursements for certain telehealth applications. For instance, a few payers may just repay live-video telehealth conferences, while others may likewise support store-and-forward and remote patient monitoring services.

- Reimbursement restrictions on supplier type also change from state to state. Qualified suppliers may incorporate doctors, advanced practice clinicians, and other licensed healthcare workers.

The American Telemedicine Association gives a state-by-state breakdown of coverage and reimbursement gaps. The territorial Telehealth Resource Centers also give data about repayment in specific states.

Worth Based Payment Mechanisms

Some provincial networks are financing telehealth programs through value-based payment mechanisms, for example, responsible consideration associations (ACOs) that value quality over a volume of care. These projects try to utilize telehealth to achieve a quality, result, and cost targets, remembering decreases for emergency clinic readmissions, lengths of remain, and transfers to larger care centers. For instance, Oregon's Coordinated Care Organizations (CCOs) get worldwide budgets to incorporate physical, behavior, and dental medicinal services for individuals. CCOs have put resources into a few telehealth activities to improve the strength of Oregonians, including telemental health services, remote patient checking, and telementoring.

Telehealth User Fees

A key element of telehealth is connecting rural sites to remote suppliers and specialists. Some rural sites contract directly with a remote supplier who can offer telehealth services. Other provincial projects pay client expenses to buy into a telehealth focus, which is regularly situated in a bigger emergency clinic or scholarly clinical focus. The expenses to associate with these telehealth services can strain offices with limited budgets. Considerations for rural programs looking to present the defense for putting resources into telehealth client charges include:

• Staffing flexibility – Telehealth allows some provincial offices to implement less expensive or more feasible staffing models. For instance, some Critical Access Hospitals may experience difficulty recruiting qualified physicians to staff emergency divisions in country areas. These medical clinics may decide rather to recruit advanced practice nurses to staff emergency departments while utilizing telehealth to empower access to remote case consultations and telementoring.

• Return on speculation – Rural people group can consider if the arrival on the venture from telehealth services justifies the expense of paying for counseling fees.

Components that may influence return on profit remember expanded income from saving patients for the network and charging for experiences. Projects may also consider cost decreases related to going for professional development and conducting recruitment activities.

• Alignment with crucial the office or organization – Some rural programs may consider how telehealth allows them to progress in the direction of the strategic vision of their association by improving the nature of care, access to care, health outcomes, or patient satisfaction.

Working with Payers and Policymakers

Some country networks may decide to work directly with policymakers, Medicaid authorities, and private back up plans to make changes to reimbursement policies and achieve long-term sustainability for their telehealth programs. Rustic projects may think about moving toward back up plans to decide whether they can utilize telehealth to achieve shared goals for improving results and decreasing expenses. For instance, a private health plan interested in decreasing diabetes-related hospitalizations may be happy to finance a remote patient observing system to improve tolerant self-management. The South Carolina Telehealth Alliance urges partners to meet with payers to offer telehealth answers for high-cost issues.

The American Telemedicine Association gives toolboxes to projects and partners keen on improving access to covered services for telehealth. Rural programs may need to build relationships with state clinical and drug store sheets to address extra factors that affect telehealth sustainability, including guidelines for licensure and certification. Rural programs may also think about joining or building up alliances to prepare assorted partners to help telehealth strategies. For instance, the California Rural Health Association was an establishing individual from the California Telehealth Policy Coalition, which creates and advocates for telehealth policy solutions.

Award Funding for Telehealth Programs

Numerous rustic projects depend on grant funding from government offices, state offices, affiliations, and philanthropic organizations to continue telehealth programs.

Federal Agencies

Numerous provincial projects depend on government award projects to execute and continue telehealth programs. The Federal Telehealth Compendium describes award funding for telehealth programs, innovation, preparing, and the sky is the limit from there. The compendium identifies telehealth programs explicit to rural communities.

State Agencies and Associations

State offices and associations may also offer telehealth award funding programs. The Telehealth Resource Centers give extra data about state-explicit assets for telehealth funding. For instance, country networks in California could apply to awards from the California Wellness Foundation, the Blue Shield of California Foundation, and the California Health Care Foundation to subsidize telehealth programs.

Foundations and Nonprofit Organizations

Many foundations and nonprofit organizations give financing or different assets to implement, grow, or continue country telehealth programs. Foundations might be keen on expanding access to mind in an underserved area, improving well-being results among specific populations, or supporting innovative healthcare delivery models. Establishments and not-for-profits financing provincial telehealth projects or research include:

• Patient-Centered Outcomes Research Institute

• Leona M. Also, Harry B. Helmsley Charitable Trust

- Aetna Foundation
- Hearst Foundations
- Robert Wood Johnson Foundation

Chapter 10

Telemedicine

1. History of Telemedicine

The field of telemedicine has changed drastically since its inception. It was distinctly around fifty years prior that a couple of emergency clinics began trying different things with telemedicine to arrive at patients in remote areas. In any case, with the fast changes in technology throughout the most recent couple of decades, telemedicine has changed into a complex incorporated help utilized in emergency clinics, homes, private doctor workplaces, and other healthcare facilities.

The idea of telemedicine began with the introduction of telecommunications technology, the methods for sending data over a separation as electromagnetic signs. Early forms of telecommunications technology incorporated the broadcast, radio, and phone. In the late nineteenth century, the radio and phone were simply beginning to rise as feasible communication technologies.

Alexander Graham Bell protected the phone in 1876, and Heinrich Rudolf Hertz played out the principal radio transmission in 1887.

Yet, it wasn't until the mid-twentieth century that everyone began to these technologies, and imagine they could be applied to the field of medication. In 1925, a spread outline of the Science and Invention magazine included an odd development by Dr. Hugo Gernsback, called the "teledactyl." The imagined tool would utilize spindly robot fingers and radio technology to look at a patient from far off and show the specialist a video feed of the patient. While this creation never moved beyond the idea organize, it anticipated the mainstream telemedicine definition we consider today – a remote video counsel among specialists and patients.

Quite a few years after the fact, in the 1950s, a few hospital systems, and college-based clinical centers experimenting with different concepts regarding how to incorporate the idea of telemedicine. Clinical staff at two different health centers in Pennsylvania around 24 miles separated transmitted radiologic pictures using phone. In 1950's, a Canadian specialist based upon this technology into a Teleradiology framework was utilized in and around Montreal. At that point, in 1959, Doctors at the University of Nebraska had the option to transmit neurological examinations to medical students across grounds using a two-way interactive television. By 1964, they had fabricated telemedicine connections that permitted them to give allowed services at Norfolk State Hospital, 112 miles from grounds.

Initially, health professionals developed this technology to arrive at remote patients living in rural areas. But with time, clinical staff and the U.S. government saw the comprehensive view – the possibility to arrive at urban populations with healthcare shortages, and to react to health-related crises by sharing clinical counsels and patient health records without delay. During the 1960s, substantial ventures from the U.S. Government, including the Public Health Department, NASA,

Department of Defense, and the Health and Human Sciences Department, drove research and development in telemedicine. Sending cardiac rhythms during emergencies began at about this time. For example, in Miami, the college clinical focus cooperated with the fire-rescue department by sending electro-cardiac rhythm signals over the voice radio channels from the rescue sites.

One particularly effective telemedicine venture supported by the legislature was known as the Space Technology Applied to Rural Papago Advanced Health Care (STARPAHC). It was an association among NASA and the Indian Health Services. The program supported remote clinical services to Native Americans living on the Papago Reservation in Arizona and astronauts in space! Projects like STARPAHC drove investigate in clinical building and extended progressions in telemedicine. The following scarcely any decades saw proceeded with advancements in telemedicine and more extensive research at colleges, clinical focuses, and research companies.

2. Telemedicine Today

Today the telemedicine field is changing faster than at any other time. As innovation progresses at exponential levels, so does the widespread affordability and accessibility to essential telemedicine instruments. For instance, not exclusively do we currently have the technology for live video telemedicine; however, a significant part of the U.S. population has experience utilizing on the web video chat applications (like Skype or Face time) and access to a PC or cell phone to utilize them.

Telemedicine was initially made as an approach to treat patients who were situated in remote places, far away from local health facilities or in areas of with deficiencies of clinical experts. While telemedicine is as yet utilized today to address these issues, it's increasingly becoming a tool for helpful clinical care. The present associated quiet needs to burn through less time in the sitting area at the doctor, and get quick care for minor yet earnest conditions when they need it.

This desire for more convenient care joined with the inaccessibility of many overburdened clinical experts (particularly essential consideration suppliers) have prompted the ascent of telemedicine organizations. Many offer patients every minute of everyday access to medical care with an available to come into work specialist contracted by that organization. Others offer emergency clinics and bigger health centers access to extra clinical staff and experts for the outsourcing of exceptional cases (basic model among Teleradiology organizations). Still, others give a telemedicine stage to doctors to use to offer virtual encounters with their patients. Increasingly, telemedicine is turning into an approach to give clinical practices an edge in a serious human services scene where it's hard to remain autonomous or keep up the main sound concern.

Also impacting the rise of telemedicine today is the growing mobile health field. With the wide variety of mobile health applications and new portable clinical devices that are buyer agreeable, patients are beginning to utilize technology to screen and track their health. Simple home-utilize clinical devices that can take vitals and analyze ear infections, monitor glucose levels, or measure blood pressure let patients accumulate required clinical data for a specialist's analysis without going into the specialist's office. Furthermore, once more, as more patients get proactive about utilizing innovation to deal with their health, they also will be more open to elective approaches to get care – through telemedicine!

3. The difference between telemedicine and telehealth

With the interrelated fields of mobile health, digital health, health IT, telemedicine all continually changing with new improvements, it's occasionally hard to nail down a definition for these terms. In a great part of the human services industry, the expressions "telehealth" and "telemedicine" are regularly utilized reciprocally. Even the ATA believes them to be interchangeable terms. This isn't surprising since the telehealth and telemedicine definitions incorporate fundamentally the same as services, including clinical instruction, e-health quiet observing, and understanding interview using video conferencing, remote health applications, the transmission of picture clinical reports, and some more.

However, if you want to get specialized, telemedicine is a subset of telehealth. While telehealth is an expansive term that incorporates all health services gave utilizing broadcast communications technology, telemedicine alludes explicitly to clinical services. There's the way the California Telehealth Resource Center characterizes telehealth:

"Telehealth is a collection of means or strategies for improving medicinal services, general health, and health instruction delivery and bolster using telecommunications technologies."

Telehealth may include more general health services, similar to general health services, though telemedicine is a particular sort of telehealth that includes a clinician giving medical services.

Here are a couple of speedy models:

Telehealth:

• A general health app that alarms people in general of a disease outbreak

• A video-conferencing stage for medical education

Telemedicine:

• A portable application that lets doctors treat their patients remotely using video-visit

• A software solution that lets essential consideration suppliers send persistent photographs of a rash or mole to a dermatologist at another area for quick diagnosis

As the field of telehealth keeps on extending and change, these terms are probably going to change and include significantly more health services.

Pursue a telemedicine demo for more knowledge into the differences.

4. Telemedicine Pros and Cons

As a rule, telemedicine is a net advantage. It extends access to quality patient care, particularly to locales and underserved populations that need it the most. It gives an approach to eliminate social insurance spending and connect the present associated understanding. It can change the healthcare delivery model for the better.

In any case, telemedicine also has a couple of drawbacks — essentially of its virtual connection, and given cultural and mechanical boundaries that could change later on. The good news is, with the developing fame and across the board acknowledgment of telemedicine, we're probably going to see the cons of telemedicine resolve themselves. With new technological advancements and moving approach that increasingly supports telemedicine, we're continuously finding ways to improve telemedicine and make it a reasonable, even invaluable type of healthcare delivery for some medical scenarios.

Here's a speedy diagram of the top advantages and disadvantages of telemedicine:

Experts of Telemedicine

- **More advantageous, available care for patients**

More accessible, convenient healthcare for patients is the main force behind the telemedicine field. Telemedicine was initially evolved in the U.S. as an approach to address care deficiencies, particularly in remote country areas. Presently telemedicine is utilized the world over, regardless of whether it's to give fundamental social insurance in underdeveloped countries or allow an older patient with mobility issues to see the specialist from home. Telemedicine has the force not exclusively to separate normal land limits to mind get to, yet to make the whole medicinal services delivery model more helpful to patients.

- **Saves on Healthcare costs**

The U.S. spends over $2.9 trillion on medicinal services each year, more than some other developed country. Also, an expected $200 billion of those expenses are avoidable, unnecessary spending. Telemedicine can cut our medicinal services spending by decreasing issues like drug non-adherence and unnecessary ER visits and making common specialist visits more efficient.

- **Extends access to counsels from specialists**

With telemedicine, clinical practice or emergency clinic framework can quickly extend access to niche medical specialists. This makes it simple for essential medical specialists to counsel clinical pros on a patient case, and for patients to see a required pro on a rare form of cancer, regardless of their area. As another model, little emergency clinics without sufficient radiology expert on-staff can outsource evaluation of x-rays through telemedicine.

- **Increasing understanding of commitment**

The present patient lives in an inexorably associated world and anticipates an alternate kind of care experience. Telemedicine draws in patients by allowing them to associate with their doctor all the more much of the time, in an advantageous way. That means more questions asked and replied to a stronger doctor-patient relationship and patients who feel enabled to deal with their care.

- **Better quality patient care**

Telemedicine makes it easier for providers to catch up with patients and ensure everything is working out positively. Regardless of whether they're utilizing a more extensive remote patient observing framework to watch the patient's heart, or doing a videochat to address medicine questions after a clinic release – telemedicine leads to better care outcomes.

For a more drawn out list of the advantages of telemedicine, see Why Telemedicine

Cons

• Requires technical training and equipment

Like most technology solutions, telemedicine stages, as a rule, require some training and equipment purchases. What amount is extremely reliant on the solution – a broader inpatient telemedicine stage that will be utilized between essential specialists and counseling experts may require all the more training and the purchase of a telemedicine truck and different mobile health devices. A safe videochat application like eVisit requires significantly less staff training and generally only requires the purchase of a webcam.

• Some telemedicine models may decrease care continuity

Telemedicine organizations that are consumer-facing offer the enormous advantage of on-request care for patients. A wiped outpatient can just log in on the web and request a visit with one of the telemedicine company's doctors and get treatment.

But, this model, like the retail health movement, leads to a breakdown in care continuity. An arbitrary specialist who doesn't have the foggiest idea about the patient doesn't have any idea about their entire clinical history. The best way to deal with telemedicine? Giving devices to suppliers to easily connect with their patients.

• May diminish face to face associations with specialists

A few critics argue that online telemedicine interactions are indifferent, and physical tests are regularly important to make a full diagnosis. If more patients are turning to online associations instead of in-person visits, what impacts will that have?

In-person patient-doctor visits are important and essential by and large. Telemedicine is best used to enhance these visits – to do direct registration with patients and ensure everything is working out positively. For minor intense conditions (like diseases), an in-person visit with a set up persistent is frequently not required. In those cases, telemedicine can spare the patient, the specialist, and the healthcare system time and money.

• Navigating the changing arrangement and repayment scene can be tricky

Telemedicine repayment is a difficult topic, especially with the continually changing state policies. Numerous states presently have equality laws that require private payers to repay for telemedicine visits a similar route as face to face visits. The ideal approach to explore repayment is to call up your top payers and ask their arrangements. You can also look at our manual for telemedicine repayment and this accommodating network from ATA on the state approach.

It's also crucial to take note that numerous specialist utilizing telemedicine will charge the patient a convenience expense, going from $35 – $125 per visit. This expense is immediate from the patient and is on (or instead of) any repayment through a payer. While that means patients are paying using cash on hand, a significant number of eVisit's customers have discovered patients wouldn't fret, and in certainty, are glad to pay the extra expense for the comfort.

5. Top Telemedicine Medical Specialties

Telemedicine is utilized in a wide range of clinical fields, all through wandering and medical clinic settings. Pretty much every clinical field has some utilization for counseling a patient or another supplier (normally a specialist) remotely. In light of deficiencies of care, constrained access to authorities in certain areas, and remote areas of patients (particularly in rustic or sparsely populated areas), telemedicine is fantastically helpful to any healthcare provider trying to grow access to quality patient care.

Some clinical fortes were early adopters of telemedicine and have pushed the development of solutions explicitly for their claim to fame. Therefore, there are a few key niche telemedicine strengths. Here are the absolute most well-known telemedicine solutions specialities:

• Teleradiology – Teleradiology is probably the most punctual field of telemedicine, starting during the 1960s. Teleradiology solutions were created to extend access to diagnosticians of x-rays. Littler medical clinics around the U.S. may not generally have a radiologist on staff, or might not approach one clock. That means patients coming into the ER, particularly during off-hours, should sit tight for analysis. Teleradiology solutions currently offer suppliers in one area to send a patient's x-rays and records safely to a certified radiologist at another area and get a fast counsel on the patient's condition.

• Telepsychiatry – Telepsychiatry allows qualified specialists to give treatment to patients remotely, extending access to social health services. Telepsychiatry is incredibly popular, to a limited extent, due to the across the nation-wide shortage of available psychiatrists, and because psychiatry regularly doesn't require the equivalent physical tests of the medical field.

• Teledermatology – Teledermatology solutions are normally store-and-forward advances that allow a general healthcare provider to send a patient photograph of a rash, a mole, or another skin irregularity, for remote diagnosis. As frontline suppliers of care, doctors are frequently the primary clinical experts to recognize a potential issue. Teledermatology solutions let PCPs keep on organizing a patient's care, and offer a speedy answer on whether further examination is required from a dermatologist.

• Teleophthalmology – Teleophthalmology solutions allow opthamologists to inspect patients' eyes or registration about medications from a separation. A typical model is an opthamologists diagnosing and treating eye disease. These plans are normally either live or store-and-forward telemedicine.

- Telenephrology – telenephrology is nephrology practiced a ways off. Telenephrology solutions are most normally utilized interprofessionally when a family doctor needs to counsel a nephrologist about a patient with kidney sickness.

- Teleobstetrics – teleobstetrics allow obstetricians to give pre-birth care from far off. This could mean, for instance, recording a child's heart in one area and sending it to an obstetrician for diagnosis at another facility.

- Teleoncology – the teleoncology field has quickly expanded over the most recent couple of years, to give more available and helpful care to patients with cancer. While some teleoncology solutions offer store-and-forward tools to advance pictures for analysis, others are live video stages to allow patient consults with the oncologist.

- Telepathology – telepathology arrangements let pathologists share pathology at a distance for diagnosis, research, and training. Most telepathology devices are store-and-forward solutions, allowing pathologists to share and forward high-goals pictures and videos.

• Telerehabilitation – telerehabilitation allows medical professionals to deliver recovery services, (for example, non-intrusive treatment) remotely.

6. What services can be given by telemedicine

Telemedicine can be utilized for a wide variety of health services. Here's a shortlist of normal conditions an essential consideration specialist may treat using telemedicine:

- Allergies
- Arthritic Pain
- Asthma
- Bronchitis
- Colds and Flu
- Diarrhea
- Infections

- Insect Bites
- Pharyngitis
- Conjunctivitis
- Rashes
- Respiratory Infections
- Sinusitis
- Skin Inflammations
- Cellulitis
- Sore Throats
- Sprains and Strains
- Bladder Infections
- UTIs
- Sports Injuries
- Vomiting

Telemedicine services can generally go by a claim to fame. A surgeon may utilize telemedicine to do post-activity registration with patients, to ensure their injury can't. A gynecologist may utilize a live telemedicine answer to giving birth control counseling. An endocrinologist may do live videochats with patients to examine late lab results and answer questions.

The list goes on. In case you as yet service about what services telemedicine is best utilized for, review this list of Medicare-repaid telemedicine benefits below. It's in no way, shape, or form a total list, yet it shows you the wide scope of health services using telemedicine that are as of now reimbursable.

7. How partners' telemedicine work/How would it be able to be utilized/Types of telemedicine

So at this point, you realize what telemedicine is. But how are telemedicine systems delivered? What kinds of technology allows digital connections between a supplier at a huge emergency clinic and a patient in a remote, rural home?

With the extension of the web, quite a bit of how telemedicine is delivered has changed. Presently, with a simple internet connection, numerous patients in remote areas can partake in probably a few sorts of telemedicine. Here are a couple of instances of telemedicine connections.

Networked Programs

Arranged associations (like rapid web lines) are normally used to interface remote health clinics to bigger health offices like metropolitan emergency clinics. As indicated by the ATA, there are around 200 arranged telemedicine programs in the U.S., giving telemedicine access to more than 3000 rural sites.

Point–to-point Connections

Point-to-point associations interface little remote health places to one, huge, focal health office using rapid web. This kind of telemedicine association lets littler or understaffed centers re-appropriate clinical care to masters in different areas inside a similar health framework. Point-to-point associations are particularly regular for telepsychiatry, Teleradiology, and urgent care services.

Monitoring Center Links

Monitoring center links are utilized for one kind of telemedicine – remote patient observing. This sort of telemedicine interface makes an advanced association between a patient's home and a remote checking office, with the goal that a patient's clinical information can be measured at home and transmitted electronically to a distant clinical observing office. These connections, for the most part, appear as web, SMS, or phone associations. They're most regularly utilized for checking of pulmonary, heart, or fetal clinical information.

8. Sorts of Telemedicine Consultations

What do you imagine when somebody says "telemedicine"? The most well-known picture is presumably a doctor consulting a patient by means of a videochat stage. Two-way video conferencing is rapidly turning into a well-known virtual option to in-person specialist visits.

A telemedicine definition includes a lot more extensive scope of social insurance services than simply ongoing clinical discussions over video. Telemedicine incorporates any clinical services gave through media communications technology. Here's an outline of the primary kinds of telemedicine.

Store-and-forward telemedicine arrangements

In some cases called no concurrent telemedicine, store-and-forward solutions empower medicinal services suppliers to advance and offer patient clinical information (lab results, pictures, recordings, records) with a supplier at an optional area. These stages offer a sort of refined, secure email stage – an approach to share private patient information online in a safe manner.

The asynchronous term refers to the way that the consulting specialist, patient, and essential specialist don't have to convey simultaneously all. As an equal, consider a call versus an email trade. A call (synchronous) requires all gatherings to convey continuously – an email trade doesn't.

Store-and-forward telemedicine works best for interprofessional medical services – where a supplier needs to outsource diagnosis to a specialist. For example, teleradiology depends vigorously on store-and-forward technology to allow technicians and healthcare professionals at littler emergency clinics to share quiet x-rays for analysis by a master at another area. Non-concurrent telemedicine is also usually utilized for Teledermatology and teleophthalmology.

Store-and-forward telemedicine is an incredible method to increase healthcare efficiency since a provider, patient, and master don't should be in a similar spot, simultaneously. It also facilitates faster diagnosis, particularly for patients situated in underserved settings that might not have the essential authority on staff. Generally speaking, this indicates lower tolerant hold-up times, more accessible healthcare, better patient results, and a more improved schedule for physicians.

Remote patient observing

Telemedicine solutions that fall into the remote patient monitoring (RPM) allow healthcare providers to follow a patient's vital signs and other health information from a separation. This makes it simple to look for notice signs and quickly intervene in patients who are at health-risk or are recovering from an ongoing medical procedure, for instance. This kind of telemedicine is now and again also called telementoring or home telehealth.

RPM telemedicine is quickly rising in popularity as more health experts understand its latent capacity consequences for constant chronic care management. For example, a patient with diabetes who has a glucose tracker in their home can gauge their glucose levels at regular intervals and transmit them to their PCP. If everything is great, those outcomes are recorded. In the case of something that looks off, the doctor may hail it and bring in the patient for a consult.

Like most telemedicine instruments, remote patient monitoring solutions make it simpler for patients and doctors to keep up close communication. Numerous RPM solutions record and transmit a patient's clinical information naturally, producing a customary report for the doctor. Now and again, this clinical information is transmitted to a group of health checking experts who are answerable for hailing any notice signs and sending them on to the doctor, if necessary.

The way to effective remote patient monitoring telemedicine is having the correct health tracking tools in the patient's home. With the recent growth of wearable and mobile medical devices, this is getting simpler. Patients have better, less expensive, more available instruments available to them for following their wellbeing signs and revealing clinical information.

Real-time telehealth

Real-time telemedicine (additionally called "synchronous telemedicine") is presumably what a great many people first consider when they hear "telemedicine." Real-time telemedicine requires a live connection between either a health professional or understanding or between health professionals, utilizing sound and video communication. Think videochat. While most ongoing telemedicine programming is substantially more refined than a sophisticated videochat stage, the essential objective is to both see and converse with the patient from a far distance. This sort of telemedicine is intended to offer a virtual option to the in-person doctor's visit.

The popularity of continuous telemedicine solutions has expanded quickly in the previous not many years, as best telemedicine organizations like Teladoc and DoctoronDemand have offered a moderate, simple route for patients to interface with a specialist from anyplace and get quick treatment.

Doctors are also beginning to receive continuous telemedicine answers to giving their patients the additional comfort of virtual doctor visits, improve their care results, support work-life balance, and receive the numerous different rewards. With essentially a perfect gadget, web association, amplifier, and webcam – a patient would now be able to get clinical treatment. That is the excellence of real-time telemedicine.

9. Telemedicine Clinical Guidelines

While the business is as yet far from a standard arrangement of built-up rules for telemedicine, the American Telemedicine Association has assembled rules for a scope of strengths dependent on a study of many research studies. What are the clinical, specialized, and managerial rules a clinical practice needs to set up when they're receiving telemedicine? Past the negligible lawful prerequisites of that state, what are telemedicine best practices?

In light of more than 600 examinations, the AMA has assembled a far-reaching set of rules for experts utilizing telemedicine in essential and urgent care. This field is quickly embracing telemedicine to extend fundamental social insurance get to. Here is a portion of the essential protocols and rules essential care or urgent care office should institute when beginning their telemedicine program.

When to utilize telemedicine

While numerous conditions not on this list can be dealt with using telemedicine, these conditions are a particularly solid match for telemedicine: Allergies and asthma, Chronic bronchitis, Conjunctivitis, UTIs, Low back pain, Otitis media, Rashes, Upper respiratory diseases, Diabetes, Hypertension, Mental illness/behavioral health, Prevention and health services.

Telemedicine ought not to be utilized for any condition where an in-person test is required in light of extreme symptoms, certain protocol-driven procedures, or aggressive interventions. Also, for a health-related crisis, patients ought to go to the ER or call 911.

Healthcare providers should utilize their expert judgment to choose when telemedicine is fitting.

When to recommend

Recommending is adequate for live-video telemedicine meetings, where the visitor can fill in for an in-person test. Prescribing is also alright for phone counsels, as long as the supplier has a previous relationship with the patient.

Informing the patient

Just a few states have guidelines requiring healthcare providers to get patients' educated agree to utilize telemedicine. But, this is, in every case, great practice, regardless of whether your state requires it. Before the first telemedicine visit, suppliers ought to disclose to patients how telemedicine functions (when service is available, booking, security and so on), any cutoff points on classification, the possibility for technical failure, protocols for the contact between virtual visits, recommending approaches and planning care with other health professionals. Everything ought to be clarified in basic, clear language.

Set-up the correct space for telemedicine visits

Healthcare providers ought to make a committed space for telemedicine visits to guarantee protection, appropriate lighting, and sound, and keep away from interferences. Whenever the situation allows, suppliers should put their camera on a level stand and position the camera at eye-level.

Make an alternate course of action for crises and referrals

Set up an arrangement for crises and share it with the patient before the visit. Make a point to have all data close by for referrals and request transfers.

Quiet Management and Evaluation

Always interact with the patient in a socially skillful manner, in the language well-known to that patient. If the patient can't understand as a result of the language barrier, telemedicine ought not to be utilized.

It is up to the healthcare provider to utilize proficient judgment to decide when telemedicine is suitable for the patient case, and when it can't. Also, the patient assessment ought to be founded on the patient's clinical history and access to their clinical record whenever possible.

To direct these choices, the supplier ought to make clinical conventions which incorporate the condition to be dealt (with ICD code), the extent of that condition that can be dealt with utilizing telemedicine, rules required to analyze (when is phone adequate, versus live video), documentation expected to review the patient's condition appropriately, parameters for when the condition can be dealt with and can't be dealt with, and rules for when the solution should be possible. While this area gives fundamental, generally speaking, rules for practicing telemedicine, it's accepted procedures for the medicinal services supplier to make more point by point protocols for each condition they plan to treat.

Required data to analyze incorporates:

- Identifying data
- Source of the history
- Chief grumbling
- History of the present sickness

- associated signs and side effects
- Past clinical history
- Family history
- Personal and social history
- Medication review
- Allergies
- A detailed review of side effects
- Provider-coordinated patient self-examination (counting portable clinical gadgets if necessary)

Quality Assurance

Healthcare providers ought to do normal quality keeps an eye on telemedicine services to identify any potential risks and failures (for example, with gear or network, and patient or supplier protests).

Billing

Suppliers ought to educate patients regarding their expense for service before the visit, at whatever point conceivable.

All in all, keep the same standards from in-person clinical services.

Suppliers should keep on observing the models they would for any in-person clinical visit. For example, they should rehearse by a similar code of morals, consent to security rules of HIPAA Laws, give appropriate documentation to the patient's essential care supplier, and follow their licensing and credentialing guidelines.

For additional details on rules for practicing telemedicine, visit the ATA site.

10. Telemedicine and Medicare

At first, Medicare just reimbursed providers for quite specific health services gave using telemedicine, frequently with severe requirements. In the previous hardly any years with the quick development in the telemedicine business, Medicare has extended the list of reimbursable telemedicine benefits yet at the same time forces numerous limitations on how the service is provided.

Here are a couple of things you should think about Medicare and Telemedicine.

- Defining the Originating and Distant Sites. Medicare repays for telehealth administrations offered by a human services supplier at a removed site, to a Medicare recipient (the patient) at an Originating Site. The beginning site must be in an HPSA (Health Professional Shortage Area). The sorts of beginning sites approved by law are:

- Physicians or practitioner offices
- Hospitals
- Critical Access Hospitals (CAH)
- Rural Health Clinics
- Federally Qualified Health Centers

- Hospital-based or CAH-based Renal Dialysis Centers

- Skilled Nursing Facilities (SNF)

- Community Mental Health Centers (CMHC).

- Note: Independent Renal Dialysis Facilities are not eligible for originating sites.

- The patient must be in an HPSA. To be qualified for Medicare repayment, the patient (Medicare recipient) should get virtual care at one of the clinical settings referenced over that is additionally situated inside a Health Professional Shortage Area (HPSA). To check whether the health facility is in an HPSA, utilize this CMS tool.

- Facility Fees. Notwithstanding repayment for the telemedicine service, Medicare will pay the beginning site an office charge. For instance, in case you're an essential care supplier with a patient in your office, and you do a telemedicine visit to counsel a doctor in another area, you could charge for two separate things – the telemedicine service, and an office expense for utilizing your training to "have" of the patient visit. Check HCPCS code Q3014 for a full description of office expenses.

• Eligible Providers. Under Medicare, the following healthcare providers can utilize telemedicine:

- Physicians
- Nurse Practitioners
- Physician Assistants
- Nurse-Midwives
- Clinical nurture pros
- Clinical Psychologists
- Clinical Social Workers
- Registered dietitians or sustenance experts
- Type of telehealth. Medicare essentially just repays for live telemedicine, where the doctor and patient are interacting continuously through secure, videochat. This sort of telemedicine visit is intended to substitute an up close and personal in-person visit. The main exemption is in Hawaii and

Alaska, where Medicare repays for store-and-forward telemedicine also.

- Only certain CPT and HCPCS codes are qualified for telemedicine repayment. Medicare has a specific list of CPT and HCPCS codes that are secured under telemedicine services. Since that list is liable to change every year, we suggest you also intermittently check the CMS site for the most modern codes.

- When charging, utilize the GT modifier. When charging for telemedicine visits, you have to incorporate the "GT" modifier with the significant CPT code to show the service was given essentially.

Discover Medicare repayment rates. Curious what Medicare will repay for a telemedicine visit? Utilize the Medicare Physician Fee Schedule Lookup instrument to type in your code and check rates dependent on your area.

11. Telemedicine and Medicaid

Unlike with Medicare, Medicaid programs are state-run and subsequently subject to state law on telemedicine practice. That implies telemedicine repayment through Medicaid is broadly subject to what the approach is in your state.

In light of the Center for Connected Health Policy's ongoing report, here's a fast diagram of what Medicaid repayment for telemedicine resembles over the U.S.:

- 46 states Medicaid programs spread live video

- 9 state Medicaid projects will cover store-and-forward telemedicine

- 14 state Medicaid programs spread remote patient checking

- Only 3 state Medicaid programs (AK, MN, and MS) offer coverage for each of the three kinds of telemedicine

- 26 state Medicaid programs spread an office or transmission charge, or both.

Things being what they are, the place do you start the examination procedure? We have 3 strong sources we use to follow Medicaid inclusion of telemedicine:

• The National Telehealth Policy Resource Center. Look at their fantastic interactive map of telehealth arrangement, state-by-state.

• Visit your state Medicaid organization site. Here's a full registry if you don't have the site helpful.

• The American Telemedicine Association. The ATA does standard telemedicine approach updates and releases quarterly reports on the state telemedicine legislation landscape. Check out the latest report here.

Components that Affect Medicaid Reimbursement for Telemedicine

Since telemedicine requirements shift by state and aren't constantly 100% clear, it's acceptable to understand what to search for. Here is a quick list of the variables you should take note of, that could influence your telemedicine reimbursement through Medicaid.

- Health Services covered
- Eligible suppliers (NPs, PAs)
- Is cross-state clinical licensing allowed?
- Is a prior relationship with the patient required?
- Location limitations on patient or supplier
- Applicable CPT codes
- Type of expense repaid (transmission, office, or both)

12. Fate of Telemedicine

There's a great deal to be optimistic about later on for telemedicine. With fast advances in technology, almost certainly, telemedicine will just become simpler and all the more generally acknowledged in the coming years. Effectively, smart glasses (like Google Glass) and smartwatches (like the Apple

Watch) can screen patients' health information and transmit them continuously to health experts. Projects like clmtrackr can analyze a person's emotional state dependent on their facial expressions and could be utilized to monitor mental wellness. Digital health startups, new businesses like Augmedix, are trying different things with naturally transcribing documentation during a patient visit. Advances in robotic surgeries allow surgeons to work on patients from far off.

To stay aware of the rate that technology is advancing, the telemedicine will need to beat other administrative barriers, for example, limitations set on telemedicine practice by state enactment, state-explicit licensing requirements by clinical sheets, and the reimbursement policies that influence whether payers and patients repay specialists are not using cash on hand. In any case, with the projection that telemedicine will be a $36.3 billion industry by 2020, more than 50 telehealth-related bills in the 113th Congress, and 75% of surveyed patients reporting interest for telemedicine,

telemedicine's future is bright, and a request is probably going to beat these barriers.

13. Telemedicine Statistics

With all the cases about the advantages of telemedicine, it is, by all accounts, an easy decision. In any case, what is the examination educating us concerning telemedicine? What do the statistics and findings of telemedicine truly appear?

All the numbers point to the exponential development of telemedicine – at the end of the day, it's not going anyplace. The worldwide telemedicine advertises worth $17.8 billion of every 2014 and is projected to grow well past that by 2020. ATA President Dr. Reed Tuckson evaluated that roughly 800,000 virtual interviews will happen in the U.S. in 2015. And health systems, doctors, legislators, and patients are fueling that upward trend. An ongoing review found an incredible 90% of human services officials were creating or executing a telemedicine program, and 84% said these programs were significant. IHS projected the number of patients utilizing telemedicine would rise from about 350,000 every 2013 to 7 million by 2018. And, with this popularity for telemedicine, legislators are scrambling to pass charges that offer both help and required regulations; in August 2015, Congress had 26 telemedicine-related bills sitting tight for choice.

The telemedicine establishment is rapidly being built. But, what's patients' opinion about telemedicine? It is safe to say that they are prepared to try it? Late examinations show that the lion's share of patients are keen on utilizing telehealth services, particularly once they perceive how telemedicine functions and the potential advantages for them. NTT Data discovered 74% of studied US patients were available to utilizing telemedicine benefits and were open to speaking with their primary care physicians using technology. 67% said telemedicine at any rate, to some degree, expands their fulfillment with clinical care.

While the loss of an in-person human association is frequently referred to by doubters of telemedicine,

76% of patients said they care more about access to medicinal services than having an in-person collaboration with their primary care physicians. Also, just 16% whenever reviewed, patients would prefer to go to the ER for minor conditions if they could rather utilize telemedicine for treatment. With the continuous lack of patient openings open with overburdened essential care specialists, these detail says a ton regarding patients' eagerness to give shot telemedicine.

While widespread research about the impacts of telemedicine is still relatively young, numerous examinations do show positive outcomes. At the point when the Veterans Health Administration actualized telemedicine for past coronary episode patients, they saw hospital readmissions because of cardiovascular breakdown drop by 51%. Another investigation on the Geisinger Health Plan indicated that telemedicine decreased 30-day emergency clinic readmissions by as much as 44%. And keeping in mind that telemedicine cynics regularly guarantee virtual visits will, in general, be lower quality than in-person visits, a recent study of 8,000 patients who utilized telemedicine recorded no distinction in care results between face to face and virtual care.

There's a great deal to be optimistic about telemedicine. A survey of healthcare executives discovered improving the nature of patient consideration was their top explanation behind implementing telemedicine. In another examination, respondents said the top advantage was the capacity to provide round-the-clock care. About a portion of patients also announced that telemedicine expands their association in treatment choices, getting them occupied with dealing with their care. Furthermore, with a potential $6 billion for each year that US bosses could save by offering telemedicine to employees, telemedicine can have a huge effect coming to past the healthcare industry.

14. Telehealth Resource Centers

The United States has 14 Telehealth Resource Centers, all supported by the U.S. Branch of Health and Human Services' Health Resources and Services Administration (HRSA) Office for the Advancement of Telehealth. These asset habitats fill in as a local hub of information and research about telehealth, generally with an emphasis on expanding medicinal services access for underserved communities. Also, the services they give are commonly free!

Chapter 11
Referrals and payment source

Suppliers to name the advantages of telemedicine, and they'll most likely say expanding access to care and cost savings. Virtual care implementations can come to the underserved, reduce no-shows, eliminate air transport, and be faster to send than new physical office space.

But revenue? That is not a typical reaction. However, numerous medicinal services leaders forget a significant revenue driver in virtual care – downstream referrals.

When referred patients denounce any authority

Referrals are a pillar of present-day medicinal services. One of each three patients is referred to as a cardiologist, urologist, orthopedic specialist, or another expert every year in the U.S. Different patients allude to essential care from emergency departments and urgent care communities. However, the referral procedure can be haphazard, including lost faxes, lost scratch pads, and inadequate EHR work processes – and finishing off with missed care.

Most suppliers additionally try to refer patients to different suppliers in their pay or system to meet the Health Maintenance Organization (HMO) or Preferred Provider Organization (PPO) requirements. Yet, 25% to half of referring doctors don't have the foggiest idea whether their patients wind up observing the provider recommended – and numerous patients pick a supplier who's out of the system or in a different hospital system, something is known as patient leakage. Patients go any authority for a few reasons:

☐ Unavailable services. Contingent upon the patient's area, the services they need may not be available at the local medical clinic. There are just 30 authorities for every 100,000 rural residents, however, 263 experts for every 100,000 urban residents. Patients requested to go hours to visit an in-organize specialist may skip treatment by and large or decide to pay out-of-arrange rates for somebody closer.

☐   Lack of telehealth choices. 74% of Millennials would lean toward a virtual visit to an in-person visit – and Generation Z is similarly as carefully inclined. Younger patients may chase down suppliers with virtual projects or even go to Direct-To-Consumer (DTC) telehealth applications, instead of going to a traditional office visit.

☐   Infrastructure delays. Indeed, even in a similar medical clinic system or association, various groups utilize a hodgepodge of technology stages and referral techniques. Patients are winding up, trusting that a referral will be submitted may strike off all alone.

☐   Online marking. Suppliers will, in general, make referrals dependent on colleague relationships – however, patients regularly look into the specialist's online reviews. They can also be pulled in by a celebrated medical clinic brand like Sloan Kettering or the Mayo Clinic or incline toward a specialist with VIP patients or a top of the line book.

Conclusion

Thank you for making it through to the end of *Telemedicine*. We hope it was informative and able to provide you with all the tools you need to achieve your goals - whatever they are.

Did you enjoy this book?

If you found this book useful, a review on Amazon would be much appreciated.

About Mike Richards

Mike Richards has been teaching in the field of medicine since 2007 using his experience gained from various institutes and training centers.
Prior to that, Dr. Mike Richards passed professional training and qualifications, and specialized in the field of telemedicine. With a unique knowledge of pulse diagnosis, urine diagnostics and extensive experience in management and cure of patients with various chronic diseases. Dr Richards has held consultations in the USA and Europe.